ON
BECOMING A
HEALTH
EDUCATOR

ON
BECOMING A
HEALTH
EDUCATOR

Gwendolyn D. Scott

Kent State University
Kent, Ohio

AND

Mona W. Carlo

Ford Junior High School
Berea, Ohio

WM. C. BROWN COMPANY PUBLISHERS
Dubuque, Iowa

HEALTH

Consulting Editor

Robert Kaplan
The Ohio State University

PHYSICAL EDUCATION

Consulting Editor

Aileene Lockhart
Texas Woman's University

PARKS AND RECREATION

Consulting Editor

David Gray
California State University, Long Beach

To Joseph M. Carlo, whose encouragement, support, and understanding made the writing of this book possible.

CONTENTS

ILLUSTRATIONS

TABLES

Table

PREFACE

Compared to societal changes education has progressed at a snail's pace. It is the intent of the authors to stir the reader to shed the bonds of traditionalism which have encompassed him throughout his own educational experiences and embrace a philosophy of change with emphasis on student involvement in learning and evaluation. Many suggestions are offered in the book as to how this might be accomplished. However, let the preprofessional understand that *these are only suggestions*. Basically, the success of any facilitator of learning rests on his accepting suggestions and tailoring them to suit the needs of his students. His challenge, then, is (1) to be creative, innovative, and excited about what he is doing; (2) to help his students to develop as total persons; and (3) to provide learning experiences which allow students to grow in self-direction.

The authors were motivated to prepare this text to help the preprofessional to assume his role as a facilitator of learning by facing in the direction toward which educational changes are moving. They envision this book as aiding the preprofessional to be able:

1. to facilitate student learning;
2. to apply conceptual models in their facilitative efforts;
3. to focus on student behavior rather than subject matter;
4. to develop meaningful behavioral objectives in the cognitive, and affective, and psychomotor domains;
5. to provide students with guidance in finding the factual information necessary for solving their problems;
6. to plan innovative learning and evaluative experiences which will actively involve students;
7. to use the technological advances in preparing or constructing teaching aids;
8. to redevelop and use their creativity; and,
9. to relate to students and their problems.

G. S.
M. C.

ACKNOWLEDGMENTS

Happiness is . . . knowledgeable consultants! From Kent State University, we express gratitude to Mrs. Ivana Cahill, who made valuable suggestions in the instructional media of the book, and to Dr. Virginia Harvey who frequently gave of her time and talent as a sounding board for developing ideas. From the Berea City School District, Dr. Dean Kelly, Mr. Neal Hesche, Mr. Thomas Yates, Mr. Richard Vale, and Mr. Neil Fort who shared their resources and many of the ideas which are encompassed in the book.

Happiness is . . . innovative educators! Much aid and encouragement were tendered by faculty members at Ford Junior High School. Particularly we are indebted to Mrs. Sharen Kinemond, Miss Linda King, Mr. Richard Brannan, Mrs. Patricia Koch, Mrs. Jane Hadden, Mrs. Diane Benjamin, Miss Carla Hoke, Mrs. Grace Stough, Mr. Robert Miller, Mr. Dale Barr, and Mr. Ted Stevens.

Happiness is . . . creative students! Since we are truly proponents of the concept of student involvement, we used as examples the products of several creative students from Kent State University. For this sharing, our thanks are extended to the following: Sue Ledyard, Lynn Hankins, Rodney Lopick, Carol Campbell, Michaela Richards, Earl Menges, Kathy Smoltz, Janet Falbo, Mary Ann King, Thomas Burick, and Ginger Hendricks.

Happiness is . . . receiving permission to cite other people's ideas! Some of the material appearing on pages 26-33 of this publication are reprinted by permission of Minnesota Mining and Manufacturing Company, publishers of School Health Education Study copyrighted 1967 by School Health Education Study, Inc. We also acknowledge the stimulation received from the writings of Carl Rogers (Houghton-Mifflin Company), Edgar H. Schein (Addison-Wesley Company), Mary B. Harbeck (*Educational Technology*), Leon M. Lessinger (*Instructor*), Benjamin S. Bloom, David Krathwohl, Bertram Masia (David McKay Company), Neil Postman and Charles Weingarten (Delacorte Press), Edgar Dale (Holt, Rinehart & Winston, Incorporated), and the American Association for Health Physical Education and Recreation.

Happiness is . . . talented technicians! Photographic assistance was contributed by Mr. Lawrence Rubens and Mr. Steven Goldman. Miss Laurel Wilcox lent her talent in reproducing several of the technical drawings, and Mrs. Lois Lehman shared her cartoon on team teaching. Their kindness and talents are appreciated.

Happiness is . . . competent typists! Our happiness was threefold—Miss Jeanne Connell, Mrs. Letty Helzer, and Miss Kathy Schuller.

Happiness is . . . an exacting editor! We express our appreciation to Dr. Doris Franklin for her skillful editing of the manuscript.

HERE AND NOW

To the college students who so vocally protest the irrelevancy of today's education, we issue a challange—make a personal commitment to change the situation!

To make sure your protests are legitimate concerns and not just popular complaints:

—Do you actually want to get involved?

—Are you vitally concerned about your prospective students and their problems?

—Are you willing to devote the time that is necessary to challenge these students?

—Are you genuinely concerned that your students have the opportunity to be involved in meaningful learning experiences?

—Can you relate to students who have a life style different from yours?

—Do you have the courage to try new approaches?

—Are you willing to risk "failures" in order to venture forth toward new horizons?

If your answers are "Yes," you *can* be an effective facilitator of change. Begin planning not what the "education establishment" should do but what you can do. The educational "system" is composed of individual classes under the charge of individual instructors. Within every school building there are classes that are dull as well as classes where education becomes an exciting experience. Which your classes will be depends on you.

The individual instructor of health education has the power and the ability to change what is often a dull, monotonous occasion into an interesting, dynamic, ever-changing, exciting experience.

The purpose of this text is to suggest guidelines that will assist the preprofessional health educator in making the transition from the commonly used traditional content-oriented teaching to contemporary concept-oriented instruction emphasizing behavioral objectives and ongoing experiences for learners.

The explosion of knowledge as a result of the advancement in medical and scientific technology is an accepted fact. The health educator must keep informed of progress in the areas related to health. To fail to do so and to be unable to guide students to pertinent sources is an indication of an inadequate instructor. Technology has made available materials and equipment that can be used with maximum effectiveness by the creative teacher.

Accompanying the technological changes is the diversity in experience and in life style of the students within a class. Experiences may range from those of the student who has had the opportunity to travel or live in other countries to those of the student whose life has been restricted to his immediate community. Some students have had extensive opportunities to associate with people of other ethnic, religious, racial, and economic backgrounds. Others lack these exposures and experiences.

Probably the most important reason for entering a plea for relevancy in instruction is the fact that issues pertinent to students are constantly changing. Thus, the students need current resources which will enable them to successfully cope with their own problems.

The teacher who desires to be effective chooses concepts applicable to student, local, national, or international issues, develops measurable behavioral objectives, and helps to provide pertinent learning experiences which can be applied to real-life situations.

Within this framework, the teacher role can be defined as a facilitator rather than as the traditional "giver of knowledge." To be a facilitator is much more difficult and it takes more skill in the planning and execution, but is also more rewarding.

With the student-to-student interaction that occurs, it is exciting for the instructor to witness students examining opposing positions, considering the implications, and forming their own value judgments. The traditional teacher tends to be so content-oriented that students tend to become less important than the subject matter. How often have we heard, "We don't have time to discuss that, because I've got so much material to cover today?" Contrarily, the facilitator is student-oriented. This does not imply that there is no "body of knowledge." Content is important as it applies to an issue or a problem. It ceases to be an end in itself to be committed to memory for regurgitation in recitation periods or for testing purposes.

The goal of the facilitator is to encourage students to become self-directing. Students must be involved in learning experiences which provide them with opportunities that make it possible to explore the alternatives available to them. Through this exploration students have an opportunity to express their ideas, hear differing viewpoints, compare the implications, weigh the consequences, and develop their own values.

When the value system and biases of the teacher are built into discussion topics, the students learn very quickly to express only the implied acceptable viewpoint regardless of the actual opinion that is held. This is known as "learning to play the game"—finding out what the teacher thinks, what he wants, and then giving it to him. This approach has worked for generations of students. But if we accept the thesis that one of the goals of education is to provide a forum where differing ideas and values can be discussed openly, is it educationally defensible to eliminate alternatives just because they are not "right" as measured by the teacher's value system?

The failure of this approach is very evident in the widespread use of marijuana and other drugs by an increasing number of our youth. One can assume that many if not most of these users have been exposed, in the classrooms of American schools, to the evils of marijuana and the dangers of alcohol.

How would you respond to these discussion topics?

1. Do you think that the possible pleasure you might get from using marijuana is worth the risk of a police record? Why or why not?
2. Should you avoid actions that will cause pain and sorrow for your parents? Why?
3. Would a good citizen report to the authorities a friend who offered him a "joint"? Why?

What astute student would risk answering these questions in the negative? These are typical closed-ended questions. The teacher is asking for specific responses and he will undoubtedly receive the "right" answers.

Contrast the above with these open-ended questions:

1. What are the current legal regulations?
2. What scientific knowledge is presently available?
3. What role does the human need to be accepted by one's peers play on the decisions you make?
4. Under what conditions do you think it is desirable to conform? Undesirable?
5. How do your decisions affect you? Your family? Your friends? Your social life? Your vocational goals?
6. What is your position on this attitude: "Marijuana is no more dangerous than alcohol. The laws applying to 'pot' are unrealistic. If I choose to use 'pot,' that's my personal choice. I just want to avoid getting 'busted.' "
7. On what basis do you make decisions?

Questions such as these put the students "in the scene" where they have to cope with making their own value judgments. Since there is no

TABLE 1

COMPARISON OF EMPHASES
BETWEEN TRADITIONAL AND FACILITATIVE LEARNING

	Traditional	Facilitative
Philosophy	Teacher has knowledge or expertise that is to be transferred to student.	Students need to develop capacity to evaluate and develop own value judgments.
Objectives	Stated in terms of what the teacher expects. Usually in cognitive domain.	Stated in terms of cognitive, affective or psychomotor behavior that the student will be able to display.
Focal Point	Teacher is center of focus.	Students are center of focus.
Seating	Formal. Teacher is confined to area—usually front of room.	Informal. Teacher serves as consultant or facilitator.
Content	Teacher-determined, dependent on facts he considers important.	Determined by those activities provided which will accomplish the stated behavioral objectives.
Source of Information	Textbook and teacher are major sources.	Multiple copies of various texts, reference books, articles, pamphlets, and community personnel are major sources.
Interaction	Teacher-student-teacher. Teacher-directed and -dominated classes.	Student - student with teacher as facilitator.
Method	Lectures, recitations, and reports are extensively used.	Problem solving that employs a variety of methods wherein student interaction is possible.
Teaching Aids	Chalkboard, films, filmstrips, tapes, transparencies, etc, are presented by teacher.	Same. Students as well as teacher are involved in previewing, developing, or presenting aids.
Testing	Factual, objective, recall knowledge.	Application of information with rationale for choices.
Evaluation	An ongoing process by the teacher.	Cooperative teacher-student evaluation an ongoing process.

"right" or "wrong" answer, it can be a frightening and anxiety-producing situation for the instructor. The teacher who needs to control the discussion will avoid this type of confrontation. What he fails to realize is that the "control" ends at the classroom door. The decisions students make are based on their own developing value systems. The most any teacher can hope to provide is the opportunity for decision-making and the opportunity to discover and use resources which can be utilized in solving their own problems.

Table 1 compares the differences in emphasis between traditional and facilitative teaching. For the preprofessional who is interested in functioning as a facilitator of change, this book provides practical guidelines. Guidelines apply to: (1) developing measurable behavioral objectives which avoid trivia, (2) generating relevant learning experiences, (3) modifying existing teaching methods, (4) creating teaching aids, (5) altering testing procedures, (6) evaluating what is occurring in the classroom and what is of greatest consequence, and (7) involving students in the processes.

2

WHY PREPARE TO BECOME OBSOLETE

It has been said that by the time a product hits the consumer market it is already in the throes of obsolescence. An interesting analogy to this situation occurs in the field of education. The facilitator, even if he has been exposed to up-to-date methodology and philosophy in his preprofessional training and does not voluntarily stay in the main stream of educational trends, may soon find himself struggling with status quo, which is, in reality, a step backward. To prepare diligently to become obsolete at the *onset* of one's teaching experience is a situation which every preprofessional can avoid, even if the education department of his institution of learning may be operating in the dark ages. How?

Perhaps one of the best means is for both the preprofessional and the facilitator to search out and observe those schools and teachers that are successfully trying new things to make learning meaningful to students. The observer might seek the answers to such questions as:

—What means is this facilitator using which enables him to reach his students?

—How might I incorporate this technique into my teaching?

To be afraid to try new methods and techniques is not just a step backwards but rather a rocket-propelled leap in the direction of obsolescence. And continued self-satisfaction with one's teaching methods is a compromise with mediocrity.

The facilitator might also keep abreast of changes, trends, and new ideas by attending workshops, in-service education sessions, and above all by reading the journals and the current books in his field. Rapping with other educators in every field and at every level can be an exhilarating experience from which new ideas may develop.

Just as the experienced facilitator must exude commitment to his chosen vocation, so must the preprofessional. One must be "sold on what he is selling" if he is to become the health educator who is constantly ahead in the struggle with the ordinary.

Health education knowledge is in a constant state of flux. This fact alone challenges the facilitator to continue his learning. He must deal with the health problems of his students in their world and must ever be alert to and willing to try new methods which will enable him to reach those in the world of today. This is not to say that every good teaching method will develop from this moment forward. Much valuable experience can be drawn from the past and bridged over to the present. But the preprofessional must accept the fact, before he enters the field, that the past is not sacred and that traditional methods need not be rigidly preserved. The world and the people in it are in a continuing state of change. Good or bad, these changes are the vehicles by which progress plunges us forward.

In these previous paragraphs various means of staving off obsolescence have been discussed. But being able to successfully reach out to kids and develop a real relationship with and understanding of them is perhaps the key to the entire teaching puzzle. It is to these relationships that the remainder of this chapter will be devoted.

Life Styles

In Chapter 1 we posed the question, "Can you relate to students who have a life style different from yours?" The preprofessional has no way of accurately forecasting what the life styles of his future students are going to be. The styles that are evolving are basically mutations of those life styles that have been labeled "American."

As we view them, there are no "pure" life styles. In each, one finds mores, ethics, values, and standards not acceptable to others within the same life style. Thus there develop subclassifications within styles labeled "right"—"moderate"—"left"—"conservative"—"liberal." As a result, the so-called liberal wing of one style may overlap, in some respects, the so-called conservative wing of another.

No useful purpose would be served in identifying specific differences and similarities between life styles. Of more importance is the recognition and acceptance that values, ethics, standards, mores held by the facilitator probably will vary considerably from those held by many of his students. In addition, the community structure has an influence on what is acceptable or unacceptable within the school setting.

What are the variations within the areas that have the potential to create conflicts between facilitators and students, students and parents, parents and facilitators, administrators and all groups?

Family Patterns. The importance of the family varies from:

1. The clannish relationship typical in some ethnic communities, to
2. The group of related individuals who get together for meals, sleep in

the same house, but otherwise rarely associate with other members of the family, to

3.   The group of unrelated individuals who form a multifamily commune for as long as it serves the needs of the individuals who make up that "family."

Male-Female Family Roles. There is a wide range in role identification, from:

1.   The well-defined role wherein father is the authoritarian head of the house, the provider, the decision maker; mother is the protector of the children and the homemaker; boys are responsible for yardwork and assisting father with repairs identified as male chores; girls are responsible for cleaning, washing, ironing and assisting mother with chores identified as female chores, to

2.   Both parents work; "major" decisions are made by father; "minor" decisions are delegated to mother; responsibilities of children may be "sex identified"—divided according to skill or rotated week to week, to

3.   Both parents work; "major" decisions are made in consultation; "minor" decisions are made by either; children may or may not be included in the decision-making processes. Their responsibilities tend to follow one of the patterns in (2), to

4.   Mother is the provider, often with a menial job; is the decision-maker and the homemaker. Household chores are often delegated to girls. Role of father may range from total responsibility for household and children to being basic nonentity.

Male-Female Occupational/Recreational Roles. The acceptance of a male-female family role will have a great bearing on the way one identifies occupational or recreational activities. This identification ranges from:

1.   Acceptance as a fact that certain occupations or recreational activities are suitable only for males, while others are acceptable only for females.

A.1.   Male occupations   Female occupations
       a.   surgeon   a.   nurse
       b.   lawyer   b.   secretary
       c.   architect   c.   hair stylist
       d.   engineer   d.   dancer
       e.   school principal   e.   elementary teacher

A.2. Male recreational activities
a. fishing
b. hunting
c. poker
d. team sports

Female recreational activities
a. knitting
b. sewing
c. bridge
d. club work (PTA, church)

A.3. Acceptable recreational activities for either sex
a. golf
b. tennis
c. bowling
d. swimming

2. Acceptance of the principle that the suitability of any occupation of recreational activity is dependent on the individual's interests and skill rather than his sex.

Religion. The emphasis placed on religion as a necessary component in one's life varies from:

1. Complete adherence to the tenets of a specific organized religious body, to
2. Acceptance of some teachings of an organized religion and the rejection of others, to
3. Rejection of any specific doctrine but the acceptance of "some higher power," to
4. Total rejection of all organized religions or of any force outside of oneself.

Language. Although English is the accepted language in American schools, there are variations unique to differing life styles. These range from:

1. English being used only when necessary. Reversion to language of ethnic origin whenever possible, to
2. The use of regional dialects, to
3. The use of colloquial expressions, to
4. The development of a unique vocabulary, to
5. The use of expressions which are categorized as vulgar or obscene by other groups.

Personal Grooming Styles. The importance of conformity to "accepted grooming standards" prevalent in the community varies from:

1. The acceptance only of individuals whose dress and hair styles con-

form to those of the community. The automatic rejection of individuals whose styles differ. The tendency to label the latter as "non-
conformists," "freaks," "hippies," or "radicals," to

2. The acceptance of individuals whose styles differ if they are considered
   otherwise "neat and clean," to
3. The acceptance of differing styles without bias.

Attitudes Toward Patriotic Symbols. The value placed on the flag
and the national anthem as being essential to the "American way of life"
ranges from:

1. Any desecration of the flag or disrespect shown when the anthem is
   played is totally repugnant and labeled un-American, to
2. The flag and anthem are symbols which no longer represent what the
   United States purports to exemplify. It is held necessary to reject these
   symbols to force recognition of dissatisfaction with present governmental policy.

Behavior. Ground rules that are unwritten but understood seem to
control behavior patterns in the different life styles.

1. In interacting with individuals who have status or authority, acceptable
   behavior patterns range from:
   a. Respect must be shown for the status figure and all directives fol-
      lowed without overt challenging. This behavior is essential to the
      adherent of "Law and Order," to
   b. Any respect shown for the authority figure must be earned. De-
      cisions and directives may be questioned. If they are seen as
      logical and desirable, they will be followed. If not, it is acceptable
      behavior to advocate a different position, to
   c. Hostility is shown for any individual seen as a part of the "estab-
      lishment." Confrontation is desirable behavior.
2. In interactions with peers, acceptable behavior patterns vary from:
   a. Conflict should be avoided at all times. Felt hostility is not ex-
      pressed. Surface politeness is an accepted norm, to
   b. Conflict can be a positive force in developing a relationship. Non-
      violent verbal confrontation is an accepted norm.
3. Interracial behavior pattern ground rules, rather than relating to one
   specific life style, cut across styles based on the racial component.
   The ground rules for acceptable behavior seem to be:
   a. Whites can confront whites.
   b. Blacks can confront blacks, but not in the presence of whites.
   c. Whites have difficulty confronting blacks. Any white-black con-
      frontative behavior will be termed "racist behavior" by blacks.
   d. Blacks can confront whites.

From an examination of the diversity of positions in the above areas, it should be obvious that the potential for conflict exists. This is especially the case if an individual in a status position adheres inflexibly to a set of values. He will inevitably find himself in conflict with individuals or groups whose values, language, and/or behavior are in opposition to his.

The preprofessional is on the threshold of a change of role—from student to teacher. With this role change will come a change in status. Thus it becomes desirable to reevaluate and identify one's own position relative to the areas listed above.

Following this identification, consider the variations of positions it would be possible for others to have in the community, in the school administration, on the school faculty, and in the student body. The problem now becomes one of determining how to develop desirable relationships with the various publics one serves. Since the relationships with the community and with the school administration are beyond the scope of this book, the focus here is narrowed to a determination of the methods that can be used to relate to students.

Reaching for the World of Students

Probably the most difficult task for any facilitator, beginning or experienced, is to discover means by which he can effectively reach out to his students because students and facilitators are so individually variable. Their life styles, values, reactions to their environment, and predictability of behavior may change from minute to minute. They may be in tune with one another or they may be poles apart. To find common ground for the development of a working relationship of mutual trust between the facilitator and the student is a tremendous challenge.

At this point the authors, rather than imposing solely their own ideas for meeting this challenge took a survey of one hundred junior high school teachers to get their reactions, asking the following "zinger" question:

"At this point in your teaching experience what have you discovered to be the best means of reaching out to students?" Here are some of the responses which may be valuable to the preprofessional to ponder:

To me the most effective technique is the personal one. If you have a periodic individual talk with students you get to know them better and to understand them better. Just a general talk about work and class attitude can give you this information. I find that talks in the halls or in the lunchroom sometimes helps as well as in the classroom—almost any time you can get the pupil alone. This personal touch seems to tell the student you are interested in him and his progress.

I've tried to use the counselors as much as possible with difficult cases and have been successful here too. The counselor talks to the students first and then we both have a meeting with him to see if we can find a solution to the problem.

"Love your enemies, it drives them nuts"—this old saying has worked for me. Just saying "Hello, how are you today?" every time you see a student seems to work with difficult cases.

I think the single most important factor is showing a student that you are interested in him as an individual, as a person who is developing and growing, maturing and learning. I think it is vital to keep in mind that in a definite sense you, as a teacher and as an adult, are helping the child form opinions and attitudes toward society and the world in general. Your attitude toward a particular student may do more to influence him than you realize. "Patience is a virtue"—trite perhaps, but true and necessary in trying to help a student *dis*cover and *un*cover ideas and opinions of his own, rather than forcing or imposing your own ideas on him. Take the time to be sincerely interested. And have a sense of humor. Laugh with the kids when they laugh and they will be more apt to work when you work.

I have found that a teacher must show a genuine interest in the out-of-school activities of the students. This includes such things as attending sporting events and praising players for doing a good job; attending dances as a chaperone; attending concerts and plays and giving special mention to the students that participated; being advisor to an extracurricular activity like chess club; being sure that a kind "hello" is spoken when a student is seen at a shopping center or movie theater; and, being able to express genuine concern for a [student's] home problem or joy for a happy event at home.

Like most first-year teachers, I have become a little disillusioned and disappointed in finding out that "reality" hinders somewhat the application of many of my more idealistic (read by some—"naive") theories of teaching and reaching kids. But much as I find it difficult to put into practice all the ideal procedures I would like to, I still try to communicate and affect my students in the only ways I now know.

What *seems* to be, for me, the most effective means of reaching out to kids is by reacting to them as one human being would react to another human being. I try to listen and respond to my students. I touch them. I try to let them know that I sincerely care about them as individuals. I try to be pleasant. Just a smile every day instead of a frown could affect students' attitudes in a positive way.

I think students' needs consist less of content found in books and more of content found in people. They need models of people, of acceptable *human* behavior patterns and responses. I have a lot to learn and I make a lot of mistakes, but for me, so far in my brief professional career, it is a simple matter of applying a very old principle called the Golden Rule.

I have found that students expect to be treated as people—human beings—not machines that are predictable. Junior high students are not predictable; therefore a teacher has to bend with them.

There are certain ways in which I expect students to behave—respect authority, be responsible, etc. And when they fail in these, I believe a teacher owes the student a bit of disciplinary measures.

I have always felt that a friendly but firm attitude is the best approach. If the students know how you feel, they usually do well in class.

Again— a student is unpredictable but a teacher should be predictable. Otherwise the student is confused.

I think the most effective means of reaching for me has been my *unconscious* enjoyment of teaching. When I reach out to the struggling masses, my personality goes first. I try to make "light" of learning. Learning doesn't have to be hard—it should be enjoyable for students. I try to get them to grasp a concept by demonstrating it with perhaps a monologue or a dialogue with myself. I clown around more than is perhaps necessary—but students have to see that *you're human*. By my dramatizing some things I am simultaneously getting more of a feel for what I want them to think about. My goal is to teach my students *to think*.

Students sometimes think I am too easy because I am willing to accept things that others won't. But to get a student to think—even one thought—is a thrill for me—and I give him credit for doing a job as best he can.

I also use my imagination to create a situation that I could apply to what we are doing. By using *my* imagination, I get them to start using *theirs*. I find that the more uninhibited I can become, the more I have reached out to them.

Some people (and educators) would not agree with my "unprofessional" tactics, but I feel that I've done a better job this year by being myself—crazy, nutty, but sometimes serious, than by being strict (super) and an ogre. By some standards I guess I'm a pushover. But I feel that I have found a way to communicate and to get my students to communicate back to me.

The only way I find you can reach kids is to be kind to them. Children of this age are so very insecure to begin with and to constantly put them down and not encourage their efforts only makes them more frustrated. Patience is a prime virtue.

I find sitting down and talking with a student about himself, his family, his attitude, etc., is the only way. The conversation must be private and with only one student; otherwise you never really communicate.

I am really not sure I know of a way. It seems that some ways work with some students and other means work with other students.

I feel that my most effective method has been to set what I consider to be a fair and *reachable* set of standards which I make clear to all my classes. I think the reason this has been successful, though, is that I bend now and then. I feel that with kids you must be understanding. Also I feel humor is a must (not to an extreme, though).

But there are days when you trust the students and they turn right around and do the opposite of what you ask. I feel that physical violence as a means of getting to students very seldom works. (Although there have been times when I have used this method, I never really feel that it has any lasting effect.)

The summary of my point: "Treat the student as a respected citizen in society."

One of the most important aspects of reaching students is to be honest with them. They must be aware that you have their best interests in mind. A teacher cannot limit his class to *his* subject matter, but must be willing to include the total education of the student as a part of his educational program.

Having good rapport with the students has helped me. They know that they will be treated justly in my class. Knowing each of their names and taking the time to find out about each one personally has helped me.

They know they can talk to me about anything and I feel that this has opened a lot of doors of communication. The men always play knowing that I, as a successful coach, care about each of them today as well as ten years from now. I hope they felt I wasn't using them for my gain but for theirs.

If at all possible I try to find out as much background on each student as possible—sports, music, drama, part-time jobs, hobbies, etc. Having this knowledge, I find it easier to communicate about subject material when I interject sidelines of interest to them.

I also feel that an informal atmosphere can be helpful, but only if the students know what the rules are and follow them.

. . . By being available to them when they need help. Treating them as human beings capable of trust and feelings really helps establish rapport.

One way that reaches many students is just listening to their problems or complaints instead of always assuming that what they have to say will be trivial.

A sense of humor is *essential*. Being fair in discipline is essential if you want to gain respect. Punishment should fit the crime, nothing too severe or nothing that would humiliate the student. If you make a threat, carry through with it.

A good teacher, I believe, is one a student can learn from not only in an academic way, but about life in general.

I have not been as successful as some teachers at forming lasting relationships with students. However, I am confident that I improve each year; and this being my third year, I have formed *some* very good relationships with my students. Probably the continuous-progress program[1] has been the main tool through which I have urged them to be more responsible. I have tried to make each one realize that they can only do as much as they *want* to do, that they must learn to think for themselves, and that they alone are responsible for their own success or failure.

. . . Sometimes I will respond to a raised hand with "Yes, sir?" or "Yes, Ma'am?" Often I call them by their last name, using Mister or Miss.

I always try to remember that the school day is only part of each student's life—often the most tedious and boring part. If there are outside pressures or worries, their attitude and performance will drop. Since many of our students are emotionally overwrought due to a very loose family structure, they are not motivated to be successful in school or in any other endeavor for

1. See page 62 for description of continuous-progress learning.

that matter. That is why I feel it is up to the teacher to make each student realize that he owes it to himself to do the best he can in all that he does. I think my students realize that I expect this of them, that I am concerned about them, and, at the same time, I respect them.

I have found the philosophy of being a student's friend *first,* then teacher *second* does *not* work with most junior high students. (At least not for me.) They are much too "friendly, forward and personal" if you let them. I find that if you joke and fool around too much they don't know how to handle it and they "take a mile." I feel they expect you to act like a teacher, but yet understand *their* need to fool around and *their* jokes.

If you attempt to add "spice" to your lesson (by a joke, comment or action) you gain their attention and many times their interest. But there is a very thin line between "adding variety" and "losing control" of the class.

Most times just a word of encouragement or a compliment (on his dress, ideas, extracurricular activities, etc.) shows the student you care. Each student deserves at least one word of "care" outside the classroom situation.

It is obvious that facilitators have many different methods which are successful for them in reaching out to their students. From these statements the preprofessional can detect that helping children to help themselves has carry-over value—can benefit them for their entire lives. It helps each individual student in developing his values, his self-image, his self-discipline, his self-restraint, and his self-concept.

Reaching students is difficult and each facilitator has to work out his own pattern as he gains experience. There are many outside influences constantly at work on each child which make him an individual. Each has an impact on his learning and achievement, the life-style he chooses, and the value guidelines he follows. The chief forces in shaping the individual, besides hereditary differences, come from his family (no matter what its structure) and the physical and social environment in which he operates. The facilitator has little or no control over these forces, but he *must* recognize that each individual is different from every other individual. It is unreasonable to believe that children *are* alike or *ought* to be alike. Inducing conformity in the classroom and teaching the masses the same content by the same method, are relic concepts of the past. No longer can the facilitator ignore the uniqueness of the individual learner. To be able to reach out and touch his students, he must first come to terms with reality and put the focus on the individual child.

Communicating

The challenge of the health education facilitator (or any other facilitator of learning) is to make education an exciting, ongoing experience for learners. Facilitating and learning in the classroom, as in any other social process, depends upon communication for its effectiveness.

To define the word "communicating" is not a simple matter. For our purposes, let us think of communicating as an art to be developed and worked at over a lifetime, the goal being the ability to relate to other people. This essential ongoing experience is not unique to education but is, rather, an inherent part of life itself. Improving communication is a key function in all education. It becomes increasingly important to the student not only in his classroom experience, but also in his role as citizen.

Communicating in the classroom is a two-way street. Unless the members of the group can communicate with the facilitator and he with them, there is very little chance that mutual trust or understanding can develop, or that collaboration toward a common objective can be reached.

As was pointed out in chapter 1, in the traditional classroom it is primarily the responsibility of the student to understand the teacher. The teacher assumes the position of *telling* students what he wants to tell them, and the students are in the position of trying to decide what the teacher is attempting to communicate. There is very little opportunity for interaction, experimentation, or challenge.

As children are growing and developing certain of their basic psychological needs become increasingly important. The needs to belong and to succeed step into prominent positions in each life. In the traditional type classroom the teacher needs may outrank the student needs. This is not to imply that all student needs may be precluded by teacher needs, for it is entirely possible that the needs of some students are truly met in the traditional classroom. However, it has become apparent, with the changes of methodology and curricula, that student-involvement in his own learning and evaluation, has lowered the barriers of resistance to learning for more students than previously. When students are given the opportunity for self-expression and experimentation without the threat of failure because their ideas may not exactly coincide with those of the leader, then their needs to belong and to achieve may well be fulfilled. There are very few situations in real life that are truly dictatorial in nature. Almost always the need is to interact and communicate with others.

All preprofessionals must ponder the problem of developing communicating skills which will adequately fulfill their students' needs as well as their own. Improving one's skill will allow both preprofessional and student to reach the intended behavioral objectives of a given concept. But just how do people communicate?

Many formulations of communication depict it as a simple problem of transfer of information from one person to another. But, as all of us know, the process is anything but simple, and the information transferred is often highly variable and highly complex. We communicate facts, feelings, perceptions, innuendos, and various other things all in the same "simple" message. We communicate not only through the spoken and written word but through gesture, physical posture, tone of voice, timing of when we speak, what we do not say, and so on.[2]

The classroom is one laboratory where the skills of communicating and relating can be practiced. However, the facilitator must have some basic concept of how to bring this situation into being. The very term "facilitator of learning" implies that the teacher no longer is exclusively in the role of "sender." The term also carries the implication that each student is involved in his learning and this demands communication and interaction within the group. "Receiving" and "sending" can be auditory, tactile, visual, or assumptive in nature. The facilitator will discover that the more these "reception" techniques are activated, the more likely it is that motivation for learning may become a reality.

How can the preprofessional build a communication system which may launch him into his career on a fairly stable keel? Let us consider negative situations to be avoided that could destroy communication, and then positive suggestions on how to help maintain open lines of communication in the classroom.

The facilitator should diligently avoid:

1. A double standard—not living up to those standards of honesty, fairness, respect, courtesy, consistency, and consideration that he demands of his students.
2. Rejection or "shutting-out" of a student by thought, word, or gesture.
3. Expecting his values and life-style to be accepted as being the ultimate.
4. Not taking the time to listen as well as to talk.
5. Setting performance standards in the classroom which do not consider individual differences.
6. Not accepting mistakes as being a part of life and learning.
7. Not considering each child as being a unique, feeling human being.
8. Planning only activities that make it easy for himself.
9. Prejudging a child from hearsay.
10. Comparing a student with other students.
11. Not attempting to understand *why* a student behaves as he does.

2. Reprinted by special permission from Edgar H. Schein, *Process Consultation* (Reading, Mass.: Addison-Wesley, 1969), p. 15.

The facilitator should attempt to:

1. Develop communication skills, have a ready smile and a "tuned-in" sense of humor.
2. Develop skill in listening, for he will discover that he, too, is capable of learning from his students.
3. Respect the thinking and ideas of students. He should encourage them to express themselves whether he agrees with them or not.
4. Understand the social environments in which his students operate and realize that external social problems overlap into the classroom. The facilitator should try to project himself into this environment.
5. Accept the reality of differing life styles and values.
6. Communicate in a language that his students understand.
7. Be flexible, kind, and respectful. He should bend again when he thinks further bending is impossible. The facilitator must realize that only by respecting can he gain respect.
8. Be supportive of students. He should communicate the attitude that even though he doesn't approve of certain life styles, he is capable of understanding. He should remind his students that the decisions they make about health practices carry responsibilities on their part.
9. Weave in statements, challenges, and concepts in the affective domain which motivate and stimulate critical thinking and discussion on the part of his students. These open the doors to decision-making.
10. Remember that each learner is a unique individual. He should be treated as such.

Gradually, the facilitator is coming to recognize that what he has to say in the classroom may not be the most important element of classroom discussion. Instead, he is discovering that two-way interactions are better and that three-way communication involving teacher-student, student-teacher, and student-student is even more effective. He must also come to understand that successful methods of communication will differ from individual to individual and from group to group. Learners in any given group may behave in a different way in that group than they do as part of another group. They also behave differently while part of a group than they behave when alone. It is the facilitator who must make the adjustment and choose communication methods which are most suitable to his situation. The skill of choosing methods is gained through experience. As noted in the foregoing responses from teachers, there are many roads to developing rapport with students. This rapport is essential to an effective communications network. As the facilitator works on his own skills, he can devise ways to assist students in improving their "listening" and "sending" skills. It is of equal importance for (1) students to communicate with each other; (2) students to communicate with the facilitator; and (3) facilitators to communicate with students.

Accountability

The preprofessional health educator must be acquainted with the "concept of accountability" which is charging into prominence in the field of education. Increasingly, school systems, individual schools, and teachers are being called to account for their performance. Just what does this term mean? The American Heritage Dictionary defines "accountability" as " . . . having to report, explain, or justify." It is simply a demand for results being issued by the public in return for the tax dollar being spent in support of education. The foremost reason for this accountability report is the rising cost of education. The public wants, and rightfully so, to receive a quality product for the money it is spending. The results it is seeking are in terms of student learning rather than physical facilities, curriculum, and yearly budget.

The authors do not propose to discuss the various proposals for accountability systems or the criteria to be used in performance measurement which are in the embryonic stage. The intent here is to acquaint the preprofessional with the trend toward accountability and its impact on the individual facilitator.

For this concept to be more easily understood by the preprofessional, he needs to be familiar with four basic terms used in the accountability concept: These are:

1. Input—which includes such items as numbers of teachers, degrees held, courses offered, space provided and, foremost, money spent.
2. Output—the student-learning results from the input.
3. Basic reforms—changes that will take place as a result of the inroads of accountability in education.
4. Performance contracting—by a contractor who agrees to improve student performance in specified learning areas, using any devices or techniques that he chooses but which are within the guidelines of the school board within whose district he is operating. The contractor is paid in accordance with the success he achieves.

The public is beginning to view the input as it would an investment in stock, property, or any other commodity from which it expects a return. Because of the pressure of this expected return all educators are having to think more precisely about what their goals are. Some teachers may view this justification of their performance with alarm. However, they must remember that if their primary concern is for growth, development, and welfare of the student, the re-examination of goals would not be a threat but rather a motivating force toward meeting the educational needs of today's children in today's world. Leon M. Lessinger states:[3]

3. Reprinted from *Instructor,* © June/July 1971, the Instructor Publications, Inc., used by permission.

Accountability can be the harbinger of a renaissance in the teaching profession . . . accountability has to do with honoring promises. Teachers, seizing leadership of the movement, will force clarity as to what they are responsible for, to whom they are accountable, and what resources and management must be supplied to make the promises an actuality. As they do so, the following will occur:

1. The focus of the schools will dramatically shift from lecturing and telling to learning, from input to output, from process to product, from time logged to competence demonstrated. Teachers will have their "babysitting" and policing functions lessened, and they will be mainly employed marshaling resources, directing learning, diagnosing difficulties, prescribing alternatives, and providing feedback on progress.

2. Patrons of the schools will come to understand and appreciate the important differences between teaching and learning, and teachers will be able to utilize a variety of nonschool resources from the media, industry, and the community.

3. The criteria for quality in education will be radically altered. Accreditation, which is now based on input, will focus on achievement as well—on demonstrated results—thus motivating communities to make teachers professionally competent.

4. The normal curve of probability as a grading standard will be exposed as poor practice. In its place teachers and suppliers will provide criterion references and performance standards, a development which will bring new authority to teachers.

5. Labeling of students as slow, or retarded, or underachieving, or culturally disadvantaged will fade as a professional crutch. Teachers will take each child where he is and help him achieve valued and clearly communicated objectives.

6. Companies and nonteachers who supply teaching materials will find, develop, validate, and offer "what works." Thus teachers will have at their command a technology of instruction including back-up training, and logistical management.

7. The performance contract will become a stable element in our schools as teachers use it to bring new and better ways into the classroom on a carefully supervised basis.

8. Teacher training will undergo drastic change. Teachers will demand competence in achieving student learning as a prerequisite to certification.
9. Salary levels for teachers will move to impressive levels as teachers are able to demonstrate results.
10. Money will be set aside to be used in developing new practices that pay off in student learning.

In the past the superintendent of schools and the athletic coaches bore the brunt of the pressures of accountability. Today the responsibilities of justification are being shared by all educators. The teachers are accountable directly to the principal of the school. He, in turn, is being challenged to develop fair and equitable tools by which to evaluate the performance of teacher and student. This may present difficulties because of the many variables which exist within any one school. Some of these variables may be:

1. the amount of money budgeted to the school (input)
2. the educational philosophy of the school, the autonomy of the principal, etc.
3. pupil characteristics (ethnic and socio-economic composition, physical influences, previous achievement records, etc.)
4. teacher characteristics (age, training, background, experience, personality, ability, attitude, the groups they teach, etc.)
5. school characteristics (size of classes, condition and age of building, availability of resources, community support, etc.)
6. the enrichment opportunities offered to students (summer school, preschool readiness offerings, extracurricular activities, learning laboratories, etc.)

Those who prepare facilitators at the college and university level play a prominent role in the accountability scheme. For example, there is very little reason why, after he has completed a health education methods course, the preprofessional should not be as prepared as any teacher in the field today to be accountable for the results of his facilitating. Otherwise, the methods class instructor is not fulfilling his contract of accountability.

This text, as will be seen in the following chapters, has preparation for accountability as one of its chief goals. It offers workable methods of planning which will enable the preprofessional to write meaningful behavioral objectives, devise student-involved activities to accomplish the objectives, and lastly to demonstrate measurable results. This, in essence, is what accountability is all about.

3

THE WONDERFUL (?) WORLD OF CURRICULUM DESIGN

As the preprofessional inspects the diversity of approach to curriculum design, is it any wonder he is confused?

A curriculum designer whose concept of health instruction is that content should be based on the learner and on the overall health problems of society will structure a curriculum within this frame of reference. One whose concept is that general health knowledge is of prime importance will use another approach. One whose concept is that growth and developmental characteristics of the young student should serve as the basis for curriculum selection will use still another approach. As an analogy, visualize a valley surrounded by mountains. On each mountain peak sits a philosopher viewing the valley below. In describing the valley, each will use his own viewpoint as a frame of reference. Which is the correct view? If there were one answer, it would be the end of all philosophical differences. So it is with curriculum design. Various designs will continue to evolve as viewpoints change. Only time will tell whether one particular design is more effective than another in attaining stated goals.

Curriculum planning and development in health education is moving from the traditionalist content-oriented model to the facilitative concept-oriented model.

The traditionalist starts with topics which he labels "units." He then develops objectives and outlines the content that fits into the unit. Thus the focus from the beginning is on the content. The content is presented to the students by various methods, using various media. The students' role is to sift out and learn the "important" facts from the content presented and be able to come up with the appropriate facts for testing purposes. The assumption here is that the more a person knows the more likely he will be to develop positive attitudes and positive behavior. To a certain extent this has occurred. Too many students, however, have developed such a negative attitude toward health classes that the potentially beneficial effects on their value structuring and their life choices tend to get lost.

Although this rejection is not unique to health education, the professional health educator has become increasingly concerned. He is aware that every day each person must make decisions that affect his personal health. Health education has the potential for assisting all students in making daily decisions that most advantageously benefit their well-being. Thus the professional health educators are searching for and developing curriculum models.

Curriculum Designs

The curricular designs commonly used in the nation's schools can be categorized according to one of the following patterns.

First pattern: curriculum determined by the textbook. The content and the emphasis are dictated by the authors. Publishers encourage the use of textbooks as the curriculum. Most publishers offer an elementary series for either the first six or the entire eight grades. Additional books are available for either junior and/or senior high levels. Teacher guides or teachers' editions, plus a scope and sequence chart, are provided. Thus textbook selection committees are encouraged to adopt a "package" from a single publisher.

Selection committees tend either to select the book or series of books that best fit an existing curriculum or to revise a curriculum to fit an adopted series. The only flexibility provided is the order in which chapters are "covered."

Second pattern: a curriculum guide for the school system developed by a curriculum director, a supervisor, or a committee representing the teachers, with the director or supervisor serving as the chairman.

The development of such a guide is frequently a summer job, which requires extra pay. Publishers are solicited for the newest textbooks and special emphasis reference books. Curriculum guides are collected from all over the country. The tendency is to "borrow" heavily from other guides—one objective derived from here, another from there, added to some developed by the committee. The same applies to content, learning activities, and references.

The resultant guides tend to be an up-dated patchwork quilt that takes its place in the "borrow from the other experts" syndrome.

When objectives, content, learning opportunities, and evaluation tools are explicitly designated to be set up within definite weeks, the facilitator is not encouraged to use his creativity to make learning exciting and meaningful for his students.

Third pattern: the curriculum guide, composed of a series of content-oriented units. The topics emphasized are those required by state edict, those chosen to "cash-in" on the problems currently receiving mass media attention, and those selected by a local group which considers them important.

This type of curriculum development is the "Let's-Jump-on-the-Bandwagon" approach. It can be shown to administrators and parents as concrete evidence that the program is keeping pace with current problems. One can safely predict that ecological problems will be the next topic to receive attention from these curriculum planners.

Fourth pattern: a curriculum developed by a group of nationally recognized specialists, which can be categorized as a proposed "ideal" curriculum. It is designed for *all* schools rather than for a particular school and is often a kindergarten-through-grade-twelve sequential program.

One of the first attempts to use a conceptual approach to curriculum design in health education was made by the Curriculum Commission of the Health Education Division, American Association for Health, Physical Education, and Recreation, which in 1967 published a pamphlet entitled Health Concepts: Guides for Health Instruction.

The Commission's concept approach[1] began with:

1. The identification of the crucial health problems of the 1960s and 1970s;
2. The consideration of these areas as they relate to health education and instructional areas;
3. The identification of health concepts pertaining to these problems or areas by well-known and recognized authorities—research and program specialists in each field; and
4. The presentation to the schools of the resulting curriculum materials leading to the concepts.

The identified concepts were organized under content areas:

Accident Prevention
Aging
Alcohol
Disaster Preparedness
Disease and Disease Control
Economics of Health Care
Environmental Conditions
Evaluation of Health Information
Family Health
International Health
Mental Health
Nutrition
Smoking

1. *Health Concepts: Guides for Health Instruction* (Washington D.C.: AAHPER, 1967), p. 4.

From the foregoing it can be seen that this group attempted to utilize the concept approach within the framework of a focus on content areas. Since it was only a listing of concepts together with some supporting data, curriculum planners could use the concepts in any way they deemed desirable.

A more sophisticated project is the School Health Education Study (S.H.E. Study). For this Study the Saumel Bronfman Foundation provided the financial support for the initial survey, the development of the conceptual model, curricular materials, as well as the pilot studies. Short-term support was then secured from the National Dairy Council, American Association for Health, Physical Education, and Recreation and the Minnesota Mining and Manufacturing Company. The 3M Company for a four and one-half year period beginning in July 1966 provided the financial support to publish the textbook *Health Education: A Conceptual Approach to Curriculum Design,* as well as the "Teaching Learning Guides" and "Teacher-Student Resources," both in booklet form, and sets of transparencies at each level for each concept.

Since the 3M support has expired, the continued development of the planned project—student booklets and student textbook series—is in doubt. At this time additional support has not been secured.

The conceptual model developed by the S.H.E. Study[2] is a hierarchical framework that defines health as "a quality of the growing and developing individual, influenced by some factors beyond the individual's control and yet directed and affected by certain choices the individual makes and executes."[3]

1. It visualizes health as having *physical, mental,* and *social dimensions.*
2. It identifies as KEY concepts *growing and developing, interacting,* and *decision making,* which are processes no individual can avoid.
3. It describes ten concepts in statement form which represent the scope of the curriculum and become the major organizing elements.
4. It generates thirty-one subconcepts, varying from two to four per concept, viewed in the three dimensions. These are the supporting ideas that serve as guides in the selection and ordination of the subject matter and in the selection and development of appropriate behavioral objectives.
5. It derives long-range goals for each concept. These are stated in general behavioral terms in the cognitive, affective, and action (psychomotor) domains. The focus is on student competencies. The goals indicate desired outcomes for the total sequential curriculum.

2. Some materials on this page reproduced by permission of Minnesota Mining and Manufacturing Company, publishers of School Health Education Study: copyrighted 1967 by School Health Education Study, Inc. *Health Education: A Conceptual Design,* pp. 15-28.
3. Ibid., p. 18.

6. It identifies a progressive sequence of behavioral objectives for each of the four levels—lower elementary, upper elementary, junior high, and senior high.

The illustration on page 28 diagrammatically depicts the S.H.E. Study curriculum model. The structure "allows for identification of additional behavioral objectives related to the concept, subconcepts, and long range goals at any given level of progression to meet individual and group differences among learners."[4]

The concepts, as such, are not taught. The facilitating is directed toward concepts that students can use in their understanding of themselves in relation to their environment. Each of the ten concepts is a part of the total scope of the S.H.E. Study model. Yet each is interrelated and all are outgrowths of the Key Concepts that are common to the lives of all.

The ten concepts are:[5]

1. Growth and Development Influences and Is Influenced by the Structure and Functioning of the Individual.

2. Growing and Developing Follows a Predictable Sequence, Yet Is Unique for Each Individual.

3. Protection and Promotion of Health is an Individual, Community, and International Responsibility.

4. The Potential for Hazards and Accidents Exists, Whatever the Environment.

5. There Are Reciprocal Relationships Involving Man, Disease, and Environment.

6. The Family Serves to Perpetuate Man and Fulfill Certain Health Needs.

7. Personal Health Practices Are Affected by a Complexity of Forces, Often Conflicting.

8. Utilization of Health Information, Products, and Services, is Guided by Values and Perceptions.

9. Use of Substances That Modify Mood and Behavior Arises from a Variety of Motivations.

10. Food Selection and Eating Patterns Are Determined by Physical, Social, Mental, Economic, and Cultural Factors.

4. Ibid., p. 28.
5. Ibid., pp. 20-23.

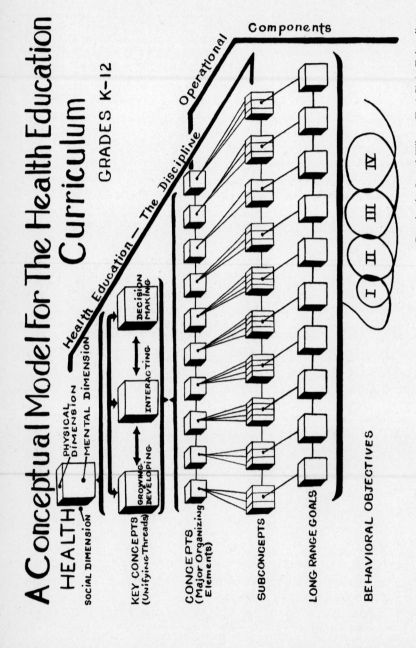

A Conceptual Model For The Health Education Curriculum

HEALTH

GRADES K-12

Health Education — The Discipline

Components

Operational

PHYSICAL DIMENSION
MENTAL DIMENSION
SOCIAL DIMENSION

KEY CONCEPTS (Unifying Threads)

GROWING-DEVELOPING

INTERACTING

DECISION MAKING

CONCEPTS (Major Organizing Elements)

SUBCONCEPTS

LONG RANGE GOALS

BEHAVIORAL OBJECTIVES

I   II   III   IV

— Drawing by Laurel Wilcox, Kent State University

What If?

The new professional will find himself in a school system that utilizes one of the preceding curricular design patterns. Thus he must find a way of functioning effectively within that framework. When the existing pattern fits his philosophy of teaching, the adjustment is easy. If the pattern is in opposition to his philosophy, the adjustment becomes much more difficult.

In a school system that has a highly structured, sequential program, the objectives and content are specifically designated. For example, a curriculum guide might designate a definite time allotment at a specific period for driver-education theory, for medical self-help, for community health, for alcohol, stimulants, narcotics, etc. The inflexibility of such a plan leaves the facilitator little room for maneuvering. Even within this rigid plan, don't be discouraged! It doesn't have to be dull and boring. The facilitator can restructure the objectives in behavioral terms without changing the implied intent and can design learning experiences that involve students.

The major disadvantage to a highly structured program is that it serves as an umbrella covering all students. No consideration is given to the many student variables that obviously exist in any school system—especially in larger cities. The guide usually does not have the flexibility for taking into account variations in the levels of learning abilities of students, or ethnic, cultural, or economic differences.

The concerned facilitator who faces the structured program that fails to meet the needs of his students may be able to push for changes by approaching the curriculum committee with the following recommendations:

1. Allowances for flexibility that take into account the variables should be built into the curriculum guide; the program would thus lose its total rigidity. Perhaps the guide itself could be organized as a loose-leaf book rather than as a bound one. In this way additions and changes could be made with relatively little expense. Alternatives could be built in that would benefit a new teacher and give him direction in dealing with his own students.

2. When the curriculum is content-oriented, it might be possible to organize study groups to examine the advantages and disadvantages of changing to a concept-oriented, behavioral-objective approach.

3. Study the feasibility of organizing experimental or pilot programs in the various schools representing the subsystems. Perhaps the S.H.E. Study model can be the basis for groups structuring behavioral objectives and learning activities pertinent to the student needs within the subsystem.

Talk to other facilitators to interest them in a thrust forward. Volunteer to help get such a move started. "Let's be innovative and let others 'borrow' from us instead of our falling into the furrow plowed by other systems." Who knows? Perhaps other disciplines may get the message and follow the lead of health education in focusing education on students and their needs.

In all the other patterns there is enough flexibility to permit creative, innovative planning within the structure.

Why the Conceptual Model ?

If the preprofessional has accepted the philosophy being stressed in this book—that the focus of facilitating is on students—he may also be able to accept the premise that the conceptual model as promulgated by the School Health Education Study (S.H.E. Study) best fits this philosophy.

The concept approach is a radical change from the content-oriented approach. The conceptual model presents a framework within which students can be encouraged to make intelligent decisions based on scientific knowledge, interacting, and on their growing and developing as well. All dimensions—physical, mental, and social—are included in each concept at each level of learning. Since the dimensions deal with the total person, particular attention can be paid to the specific needs of individual students.

Weaknesses of the Conceptual Model

As might be expected, no curriculum design has been developed that is flawless.

The S.H.E. Study design purports to weave the mental-emotional design throughout each concept. It does the same with the physical and social dimensions. Yet all ten concepts focus attention on the physical or social aspects of health. Thus mental-emotional aspects are ignored in structuring the concepts.

A second problem is not a flaw in the design, but rather an organizational reality that faces the professional. The S.H.E. Study curriculum is very comprehensive. It has been designed for ideal circumstances where health education is offered on a regular basis, K-12, to all students. Rarely will the preprofessional find himself in such a utopian set-up. It is more realistic for him to discover that health education will be offered once or twice at the junior high level for one or two periods on either a semester or full year basis. At the senior high school level, the common patterns range from no health education, to a one-semester course of five days per week or a two-semester course of two days per week. Thus to plan to implement a curriculum as extensive as that which the S.H.E. Study presents would be unrealistic.

A third problem area involves the expense of adopting the S.H.E Study "package." As noted earlier, visuals in the form of series of transparencies for each concept and at each level have been prepared. The quality and potential usefulness of many of the individual visuals is questionable. Yet it is not possible to purchase the transparencies individually. Originally masters were provided so that copies of the ones deemed valuable could be reproduced. Subsequent elimination of the masters made selective reproduction impossible.

Whenever teaching aids are prepared for use by other professionals, the problem of personal evaluation arises. What one person finds useful, another may reject as useless.

Even if all visuals in the Study package were deemed valuable, it is questionable, in view of the scheduling realities and the financial situation of the schools, whether such an expense for a single type of teaching aid can be justified. The funds that would need to be expended might be better used on a variety of media. Any medium which is overused tends to lose its effectiveness.

Utilizing the Conceptual Model

Even though the S.H.E. Study curriculum is no panacea, it is still the best design for the student-oriented philosophy.

To offset the lack of focus on the mental-emotional aspect, one might develop and add an eleventh concept. Consider this as a possibility:

Emotional health is influenced by interpersonal relationships and enhanced by an understanding of the factors affecting behavior.

The physical, social, and mental dimensions can be defined, subconcepts developed, and behavioral objectives formed which apply to one's students.

Given the framework within which the facilitator must function, it is conceivable that he can still design his program within the confines of the S.H.E. Study. If he is free to determine the concepts to be dealt with in the school year (that is, if he is not locked into a prescribed curriculum designed for an entire school system), he has possibly two alternatives he may consider.

1. He may make the concept choices based upon
    a. the past health learning experiences of his students,
    b. the needs of his students as he views them, and
    c. the requirements of his school system and the state in which he teaches.

2. He may involve his students in choosing the concepts that they feel would be of greatest value to them. Thus they might well filter out any learning areas that have been overexposed. This involvement alternative also places a degree of responsibility for learning upon the students from the start. Consider the following tabular example of how this student selection of concepts might be accomplished:

Student Choices of Concepts

Directions—All health education knowledge can be classified within eleven concepts.[6] Listed below are these eleven concepts and a brief description of what is involved in the learning of each. Choose three of the concepts which interest you the most and which you feel are important to you at this stage in your growth and development. Indicate your choices by placing a check in the left column.

Check Here

1. Growth and Development Influences and Is Influenced by the Structure and Functioning of the Individual.
    Learning involvement: Heredity, body functions, environmental conditions, and other factors which may hinder or promote growth and development.

2. Growing and Developing Follows a Predictable Sequence, Yet Is Unique For Each Individual.
    Learning Involvement: Individual differences in growing and developing influenced by heredity, environment, and personal practices.

3. Protection and Promotion of Health is an Individual, Community, and International Responsibility.
    Learning involvement: Everyone's responsibility for safeguarding, maintaining, and promoting his own health, that of his community, country, and the world.

4. The Potential For Hazards And Accidents Exists, Whatever the Environment.
    Learning involvement: Respecting the possibility that accidents and hazards may occur whenever the human factor is introduced into an environment.

6. Based upon the ten concepts appearing on pp. 20-23, the S.H.E. Study.

5. There Are Reciprocal Relationships Involving Man, Disease, and Environment.
   Learning involvement: Health status as influenced by man's effect upon the environment, and the environment's effect upon man.

6. The Family Serves to Perpetuate Man And Fulfill Certain Health Needs.
   Learning involvement: Reproductive education, human sexuality, responsibilities of family members for fulfilling the basic emotional, physical, and social needs of one another.

7. Personal Health Practices Are Affected by a Complexity of Forces, Often Conflicting.
   Learning involvement: The choices a person makes regarding his own health practices influenced by physical, mental, and social factors.

8. Utilization of Health Information, Products, and Services, Is Guided by Values And Perceptions.
   Learning involvement: Values of the individual that guide his choice of the information he wishes to internalize, the health products he will use, and the health services he will seek.

9. Use of Substances That Modify Mood and Behavior Arises From a Variety of Motivations.
   Learning involvement: Motivations of people to become nonusers, users, and misusers of substances that change feelings and behavior.

10. Food Selection and Eating Patterns are Determined by Physical, Social, Mental, Economic, and Cultural Factors.
    Learning involvement: Considers nutrition education, the influence of balanced diet on growing and developing physically, mentally, and socially, and the environmental influences on food choices.

11. Emotional Health is Influenced by Interpersonal Relationships and Enhanced by an Understanding of the Factors Affecting Behavior.
    Learning involvement: Considers basic emotional needs of all people, who supplies these needs, and how the lack of fulfillment of one or more leads to changes in behavior.

The facilitator may use as many student choices of concepts as he can fit into his planning for the year, in the priority that the students indicate. It is obvious that, in most cases, eleven concepts cannot be adequately dealt with in a single year.

Even if the facilitator chooses to use the conceptual model as set forth in the S.H.E. Study, he may possibly discover that some of the subconcepts described therein do not particularly suit the needs of his own students. If this is the case, there is no reason why he cannot develop subconcepts of his own that will take into consideration:

1. The various ethnic, cultural, and economic subgroups within his school;
2. The particular health problems present within the society in which his students coexist; and
3. Their previous learning experiences.

Again, in developing these subconcepts the facilitator may wish to involve his students. The following table presents an example of how this might be done:

Student Involvement in Developing Subconcepts

Directions: Most of you have studied some phases of the concept "The Family Serves to Perpetuate Man and to Fulfill Certain Health Needs." Your reaction to some of the content areas that should be emphasized this year will help your teacher(s) in devising the program that will be most interesting and meaningful to you. If you feel that a particular part should be dealt with, circle letter "A" in the margin. If you think the problem is interesting but should not be pursued in this health education class, circle letter "B." If, in your opinion, the subject is not interesting or if you have dealt with it enough in previous classes, circle letter "C."

A—Should be stressed.

B—Interesting, but should not be dealt with in this health education class.

C—Not interesting.

1.	A	B	C	Factors that contribute to successful family living.
2.	A	B	C	Family fragmentation (factors that destroy a family).
3.	A	B	C	The changing male/female roles.
4.	A	B	C	Human sexuality, deviations.

5.	A	B	C	Reproduction education.
6.	A	B	C	The problem of overpopulation.
7.	A	B	C	Responsibilities in dating, the stages of love.
8.	A	B	C	Choices: Marriage (mate selection), career, or both.
9.	A	B	C	Problems of early marriage.
10.	A	B	C	Differences between families (cultural, religious, economic values).
11.	A	B	C	Problems of the aged.
12.	A	B	C	The impact of nutrition on children.

After the facilitator gets an indication of the areas of student interest within a given concept, he can develop them into subconceptual statements. He may then inspect the suggested behavioral objectives, eliminate those that don't apply, develop those that are applicable to his students, and devise suitable learning experiences pertinent to the objectives. Again, he may choose to involve his students in setting the learning objectives. How might this be done?

1. The students may be given a list of facilitator-prepared learning objectives, from which they are given the option of choosing those important to them; or
2. The students may be actively involved in designing the objectives.

If the second method is chosen, the facilitator must:

1. Have students discuss what an objective is and why objectives are a necessary part of learning; and
2. Show students that learning objectives, in order to be reached successfully, must describe
    a. who is to perform the action,
    b. what the specific action or ability is,
    c. how it is to be done,
    d. with what degree of efficiency the action is to be carried out (can the action be measured?).

It may be surprising to the preprofessional, who struggles with the transfer from *teaching* objectives to *learning* objectives, that the students he teaches may very well be able to develop this skill.

Regardless of the type of curriculum model chosen by or imposed upon a facilitator, the responsibility for making learning in health education an exciting, meaningful experience rests upon his shoulders. If the subject, in the mind of the teacher, is a "step-sister" to some other interest area, or if he demonstrates a "ho-hum" attitude, he will surely kill learning. The inferior teacher can take a potentially effective curriculum, move mechanically through it, and utterly destroy that potential.

The key to *any* successful curriculum manifestation is the superior teacher who:

1. Can make the classroom come alive;
2. Feels free to experiment;
3. Involves his students;
4. Challenges students to think, seek, and discover;
5. Gives students the opportunity to make self-conceived decisions;
6. Sees his role as facilitating growth in *each* student;
7. Displays enthusiasm and eagerness; and
8. Is "sold on what he is selling."

For the preprofessional who has been brainwashed into believing that the factual information he has gathered throughout his career is the most important of his equipment, it can be traumatic to realize that his personality, the way he relates to his students, and his becoming a superior teacher will have a greater impact on the students whose lives he touches than will the content of what he teaches.

4

ALL FACILITATORS: TAKE ONE STEP FORWARD

The expectation of the facilitative health educator is to activate inert interests. He wants to share with his students the excitement and fascination of the concepts of healthful living. If he is successful, students will apply the concepts in their continuing struggle for self-actualization. Through involvement in the learning activities, they will be encouraged to develop their comprehension, enticed to display positive attitudes based on their understanding, and encouraged to improve their sensitivity to others' points of view.

These purposes cannot be achieved without careful planning. Past experience has shown us that health concepts cannot be inflicted successfully upon our youth. Unless students accept healthful living as a desirable, relevant goal, they will continue to view health education as a minor, unimportant, nonrelevant requirement imposed to enable them to graduate.

As previously mentioned, the facilitative model focuses on students. Thus, the facilitator, to accomplish his goals, must gather some basic data relative to his students, their school, and their community. He needs to contact school and community resources to find answers to pertinent questions: (1) What are the major health problems in the school? In the community? (2) What are the areas of instruction required by law? (3) What is dictated by the school system via a curriculum guide? (4) What resources are available within the school system? (5) What governmental, voluntary, professional, or commercial agencies are located in the community? (6) What information is available from the prior instructor's records that provides insights into the previous health education experiences of the students he will have?

After compiling this information, the health educator selects pertinent concepts and subconcepts and tentatively blocks these into time segments in the school year.

Now comes one of the highest hurdles that the inexperienced facilitator faces—the development of instructional objectives for each concept.

Constructing meaningful instructional objectives has always been a difficult chore for most preprofessional students. Theoretically the objectives were to be developed as the initial step in planning the resource unit, the teaching unit, or the individual lesson plan. Actually what often occurred was that units or plans were developed first. The content was inspected and objectives were added on the basis of what the teacher planned to cover. Thus objectives were normally stated in terms of (1) what the teacher planned to accomplish, (2) student knowledge or understanding, or (3) learner behavior in broad general terms.

The classification scheme presented in the *Taxonomy of Educational Objectives* has been instrumental in focusing objectives on the competencies exhibited by the learner rather than on the content presented. These objectives indicate a specific behavior change in the learner due to a change in knowledge, attitudes, values, or skills.[1]

Statements that describe observable actions or abilities, that may give the circumstances under which the performance occurs, that contain content, and that provide a means of confirming success are called *behavioral objectives*.

Although some educators oppose the use of behavioral objectives, there are several advantages which shouldn't be overlooked. Behaviorally stated objectives provide guidance to the instructor in structuring the learning experiences. He knows what type of activities to plan to enable students to exhibit the stated behavior. He is directed to the content which must be supplied. He receives guidance as to the method necessary to evaluate success. In addition, when behavioral objectives are shared with students, the purpose of the instruction tends to be clearer.

There are several ways these objectives may be communicated to students. Either they may be spelled out on a guide sheet given to each one at the beginning of a concept for constant reviewing; they may be projected on a transparency from the overhead projector; they may be written on the blackboard; or, in the case of a large group lecture the learning objectives for the lesson may simply be stated verbally at the beginning. The students know what they are to accomplish, under what circumstances, and whether or not they are successful.

Bloom's *Taxonomy*[2] provides a system whereby all educational objectives can be structured in terms of measurable behaviors and classified in the cognitive domain, in the affective domain or in the psychomotor domain.

A general understanding of the three domains is necessary before valid behavioral objectives can be constructed.

1. Benjamin S. Bloom, David R. Krathwohl, and Bertram Masia, eds. *Taxonomy of Educational Goals: Cognitive Domain* and *Affective Domain,* 2 Handbooks (New York: David McKay Co., Inc. 1956-64).
2. Ibid.

Cognitive Domain

"The cognitive domain includes those objectives which deal with recall or recognition of knowledge and the development of intellectual abilities and skills."[3]

The taxonomy is arranged in six major classes which move from the simple to the complex; from the concrete to the abstract:

1. Knowledge
2. Comprehension
3. Application
4. Analysis
5. Synthesis
6. Evaluation

Knowledge (the lowest level)—Involves the recall of specific factual information.[4]

Comprehension—Involves knowing what is being communicated, either in oral or written mode. There is an assumption that some use of the ideas can be made.[5]

Application—Involves the ability to recall the appropriate idea, theory, or principle and to use the abstraction in a particular situation.[6]

Analysis—"Emphasizes the breakdown of the material into its constituent parts, . . . the detection of the relationships of the parts, or . . . the techniques and devices used to convey the meaning . . . of a communication."[7]

Synthesis—Involves the combination of the component parts " . . . in such a way as to constitute a pattern or structure not clearly there before."[8]

Evaluation—Involves quantitative or qualitative judgments. The use of standards or criteria to measure the accuracy, effectiveness or value of something—an idea, a solution, a product.[9]

If one were to inspect the stated objectives of most educators, the majority of them would fall in the cognitive domain and in the knowledge or comprehension classifications. Thus, in health education, the learner has been expected to recall or recognize facts in isolation. Health educators have frequently emphasized the specific parts of the anatomical structure and physiological functions. Some instructors have made concerted efforts to have students apply the facts to their lives. As one inspects teacher-made

3. Bloom, et al., *Taxonomy*, Handbook I: *Cognitive Domain*, p. 7.
4. Ibid., p. 62.
5. Ibid., p. 89.
6. Ibid., p. 120.
7. Ibid., p. 144.
8. Ibid., p. 162.
9. Ibid., p. 185.

tests, however, the test items are invariably of the recall variety that fit so well into objective-type tests. Here the content rather than the learner receives the emphasis.

Behavioral objectives which can be classified in the cognitive domain are important and are necessary. For a facilitator to develop significant instructional objectives, he needs to focus on the students and determine:

1. What behaviors or competencies are essential for them to function effectively in their world?
2. What competencies will it be possible for learners to develop within the time framework provided (class period, week, month, etc.)?
3. What competencies are the students capable of exhibiting which are at a higher level than the lowest classification?
4. What specific behaviors can be exhibited which will provide observable or measurable methods for evaluating successful accomplishment?

Facilitators need to recognize the importance and desirability of the other domains. One cannot be satisfied with limiting the students' competencies to the cognitive domain.

Affective Domain

The affective domain includes those objectives which emphasize values, interests, attitudes, emotions, or feelings. Again there is a hierarchial arrangement of classes from the simple to the complex; from the concrete to the abstract:

1. Receiving
2. Responding
3. Valuing
4. Organization
5. Characterization by a value or value complex

Receiving—Involves being able to recognize, being conscious of, or being able to tolerate phenomena or stimuli.[10]

Responding—Involves a range of reaction from passive compliance through voluntary willingness, to actively receiving a feeling of pleasure or enjoyment from the response.[11]

Valuing—Involves a range of acceptance each step of which represents a stage of deeper internalization: that a thing, phenomenon, or belief has worth; that one is sufficiently committed to the value to want it or to pursue it; that one is committed to the degree of "holding the value."[12]

10. Bloom, Krathwohl, et al., *Taxonomy*, Handbook II: *Affective Domain*, pp. 98-108.
11. Ibid., pp. 118-31.
12. Ibid., pp. 139-50.

Organization—Involves an organizational system for values pertaining to situations where more than one value is pertinent: (a) conceptualization which includes determining commonalities as well as differentiation; (b) determination of the interrelationships of the values; (c) establishment of dominant values.[13]

Characterization by a value or value complex—Involves consistent behavior in accordance with a system of accepted values; the integration of beliefs, ideas, and attitudes into a total philosophy of life.[14]

Learning to make value judgments and to build value systems is one of the bridges to a more complete education—to more effective living. Health education has the opportunity to aid students in growing in this direction.

If learning in health education is to be relevant to the student, it must be laced with value education. Everyone cannot be cast into the same mold in the acceptance of health values. But every student should have some minimal acceptance level to which he adheres. From here, then, it is hoped that, through exposure, further personal growth will take place.

Measurable objectives can be devised in health education such as will allow the student to exercise his ability to make judgments, to fortify his existing values, or to rearrange his own preferences. This affective learning domain, which, because of its nebulous nature, has been ignored or avoided by most educators, is the one health educators should seize upon, develop, and utilize to the utmost. What better medium is there in the entire educational expanse than health education for the employment of educational objectives in the affective domain? What better opportunities are present for lively discussions between students with different cultural and spiritual backgrounds, value systems, and appreciations than in the health education classes? Individual differences in character and personality result in a great diversity of acceptable behaviors in response to given circumstances.

To be sure, it is more difficult to pose objectives in the affective domain than in the cognitive domain. In the cognitive behaviors the student demonstrates his intellectual capabilities, which are readily measurable. In the affective domain he shows, through his behavior, what he is thinking or feeling. No teacher should be afraid to attempt to measure in some way a student's ability to make value judgments and defend them. Even though this type of learning and behavioral outcomes may seem "hairy" for the facilitator, it is a great step forward in making learning more meaningful to the student.

It is our premise that the goals of the facilitator are to assist students to become more self-assured, more self-determined, more understanding

13. Ibid., p. 154.
14. Ibid., pp. 165-71.

of others, and to value themselves more highly than they did prior to the
onset of the experience. If these fail to occur or the climate which permits
these to take place is missing, the facilitator fits the "traditional model"
rather than the "facilitator model."

Although Carl Rogers, in his writings, referred to learning in reference to psychotherapy, it is quite conceivable that the outcomes he defines should also be desirable within the educational experience.

1. The person comes to see himself differently.
2. He accepts himself and his feelings more fully.
3. He becomes more self-confident and self-directing.
4. He becomes more the person he would like to be.
5. He becomes more flexible, less rigid in his perceptions.
6. He adopts more realistic goals for himself.
7. He behaves in a more mature fashion.
8. He changes his maladjustive behaviors . . .
9. He becomes more acceptant of others.
10. He becomes more open to the evidence, both to what is go-
    ing on outside of himself, and to what is going on inside of
    himself.[15]

The health educator cannot possibly or rightfully assign a grade to a
student for his interests, values, choices, or judgments. But he can construct affective objectives which are measurable and can be evaluated. Also
he has the opportunity to make astute observations of the student's health
behaviors in and out of school. The facilitator is usually aware to some
extent of the student's (1) choice of reading materials in the library or
study halls, (2) use or nonuse of tobacco, (3) observable relationships with
the opposite sex, (4) interest in physical activity, (5) absences from
school, (6) food selection at lunch, (7) abrupt changes in behavior, (8)
tensions or laxity, (9) willingness to work above and beyond the requirement, (10) participation in discussion groups, (11) initiation of ideas,
(12) creativity stimulated by interest and appreciation, (13) choice of
friends, (14) language usage, (15) personal grooming habits, (16) use of
leisure time, (17) conformity or nonconformity to rules, and many other
demonstrable affective behaviors. All of these overt behaviors can indicate whether the student is on his way to developing a value system, and an
adequate self-image—which need *not,* incidentally, conform to the teacher's criteria of adequate values.

15. Carl L. Rogers, *On Becoming a Person* (Boston: Houghton Mifflin Co., 1961),
p. 280.

The teacher must not be deceived into thinking that because the student is "aware" or "appreciates," he is necessarily going to incorporate these behaviors into his living style. In this affective domain, what a student *knows* and what he *does* may be two different things. But the circumstances must be present for the student to have a choice. An example is smoking. Most young people are fully "aware" of the immediate and long-range effects. Yet, because of personal needs or pressures of an immediate nature, many are still deciding to begin smoking or to continue smoking.

The affective domain cannot be ignored, regardless of the difficulties encountered. Teachers *do* show values and students *do* develop values. Often what a teacher *does* speaks louder than what he *says*. It seems safer to continue to consciously work on evaluation in this area than to leave it to chance and hope for the best. The affective domain is central to every part of the learning and evaluation process. Awareness initiates learning. Willingness to respond is the basis for psychomotor responses, and value systems provide the motivation for continued learning and for most of the individual's overt behavior.[16]

In a world of "do your own thing" blind conformity, in theory, is "out." If any person, and the student in particular, is to do his own "thing" then he has to be capable of understanding what his "thing" is. One does not wave a magic wand, or pop a super pill and have an instant "thing" to do. "Things" have to evolve from "things," things like interactions, experiences, and knowledge. In order to pursue the "things" he wishes, it is obvious that the student must be capable of making value judgments and develop appreciations. Situations that will cause the student to receive, respond, and evaluate can be devised by the teacher through the use of behavioral objectives written in the affective domain.

Psychomotor Domain

The psychomotor domain includes those "objectives which emphasize some muscular or motor skill, some manipulation of materials and objects, or some act which requires neuromuscular coordination."[17]

Objectives written in this domain will receive the most emphasis in classes that focus on the development of a motor skill, such as home economics, industrial arts, physical education, art, or music. This should not be interpreted as meaning that objectives in the psychomotor domain

16. Mary B. Harbeck, "Instrumental Objectives in the Affective Domain," *Educational Technology,* January, 1970, p. 150.
17. Bloom, Krathwohl, et. al., *Taxonomy,* Handbook II: p. 7.

should be rejected by the health educator. Perhaps, in contrast, objectives in this domain should be utilized to a greater degree. Learning objectives in this domain make use of physical behaviors as an observable, measurable expression of knowledge or values. The imaginative teacher will be able to devise and employ a variety of meaningful behavioral objectives in the psychomotor domain.

The behaviors could be in the form of demonstrations, laboratory type activities, sociodramas, nonverbal expressions (mimicry, charades), constructions, manipulative actions, compositions (music, lyrics, dance, or poetry) which can be performed, slogans, cartoons, charts, and numerous other motor activities.

It must be apparent to the preprofessional, at this point, that there is a great interrelationship and much overlapping between the three domains. What makes the subtle differences between the three is where the focus is placed—on intellectual outcomes, on feeling or emotional outcomes, or motor skill outcomes. It can be pointed out that objectives of the psychomotor domain usually include elements from both the cognitive and the affective domains. As an example, a learner may desire to improve a demonstrated skill (affective or psychomotor). In order for this improvement to take place he may have to learn more about what is involved (cognitive). To be outstanding in the execution of the skill he must practice conscientiously (psychomotor).

Formulating Behavioral Objectives

Behavioral objectives are termed *behavioral* because they contain content and an expected behavioral change in the learner that can be demonstrated, observed, and measured. When properly stated, these changes can take place in his thinking, in his feelings, or in his actions.

The use of behavioral objectives can unlock the teacher's imagination and can help him to utilize multi-media in facilitating student learning. These types of experiences are more meaningful to the learner. Reduced is the type of boredom where the student is present in body but not in mind.

Often it is difficult for a teacher to transfer his thinking from the *self-centered* teaching objectives to *student-centered* learning objectives. Now, rather than the phrase, "My objective is . . . ," he begins to think, "The student will be able to . . . ."

The task of transferring one's thinking to this direction is often a stumbling block to an experienced teacher. The prospective teacher who initially develops this technique of planning has a distinct advantage.

Of potential value to the preprofessional educator is Postman and Weingartner's *Teaching as a Subversive Activity*. They see the facilitator as "an inventor of viable new teaching strategies" and suggest that the teacher "Write on a scrap of paper these questions:

What am I going to have my students do . . .?
What's it good for?
How do I know?[18]

We suggest that facilitators keep these in mind while pondering the following additional questions in relation to each concept:

1. What competencies within this concept should the student achieve that are relevant to his world?
2. What experiences can be provided to enable him to develop these competencies?
3. How can his performance be evaluated?

After considering these questions, the facilitator will be able to see that his success in solving them will rest upon his ability to formulate objectives describing some development of the learner.

The content of an objective can be of either a general or a specific nature.

If the objective is stated in general terms, it is designed to have many possible outcomes. The general behavioral objective is normally used in a resource unit or in a teaching unit. It has no behavior stated in observable or measurable terms. The content is also defined in broad terms. The following is an example of a general objective. Note that the phrase "The student is able" is understood and need not be stated.

(The student is able) to recognize the behavioral changes that may occur in a drug abuser.

As can be seen, the specific behavior that will demonstrate the ability "to recognize" is absent. In addition, the term "drug abuser" is also general and thus could include any drug from aspirin to ZNA. ZNA is a mixture of dill weed and monosodium glutinate which is smoked for alleged hallucinogenic effects.

There is a simple rationale for omitting the specific details in these objectives:

1. If all the possible drugs were named, the listing of objectives would be endless.
2. The flexibility enabling one to include or exclude various drugs dependent on the relevance to a particular group of students, is built-in.
3. There is flexibility for a determination of what observable behavior is desired relative to the skills of a specific group of students.

Specific behavioral objectives are most useful in planning for individual lessons. At this point, the facilitator has a particular group of stu-

18. Neil Postman and Charles Weingartner, *Teaching as a Subversive Activity* (New York: Delacorte Press, 1969), p. 193.

dents about each of whom he has some information. He knows whether they need to develop their verbal, written, or motor competencies. He knows whether they need more experience in manipulating concrete or abstract concepts. Thus he can structure a behavioral objective to provide the type of experience needed.

When formulating specific behavioral objectives in any of the domains, the facilitator needs to remember that they are written in terms of the learner and:

1. Are related to a general objective;
2. Describe a specific action or ability;
3. May state the circumstances under which the performance occurs;
4. Contain content drawn from the concept;
5. Are measurable through pretesting immediate recognition or post evaluation.

Analyze the following objective. Does it meet the above criteria?

Through small group discussion, students will be able to generate a written list to identify three physical, or three emotional, or three social behavioral changes which may occur in an abused of barbiturates (downers).

Upon examination, it can be noted that the specific objective (1) is related to the previously stated general objective; (2) designates working in a small group for the circumstances under which the performance occurs; (3) focuses on a particular group of drugs—"downers"; and (4) the written list can be evaluated immediately if the results are verbally fed back to the total class. If not, the written lists can be evaluated at a later time. The new teacher developing the ability to write behavioral objectives finds that everything falls into place because he has every phase of his planning mapped out. He knows what learning activities must be provided in order for the learner to accomplish the objective. He also knows that the student's performance can be measured. But a word of warning: if the objective is not measurable, there will be no way for the teacher or the student to determine whether it has been achieved successfully.

Tailoring Objectives for Each Domain

At this point, let us examine how the facilitator can tailor specific behavioral objectives in each of the domains.

The cognitive domain, as previously mentioned, encompasses facts and intellectual manipulation. Assume that this is a general objective in the concept with which the facilitator is dealing:

(The student is able) to analyze the factors that affect food selection patterns.

A sequential series of specific behavioral objectives can be planned to enable the students to accomplish the above objective.

1. When given a list of food prices and a list of foodstuffs purchased by families consisting of four members, and representative of poverty-level, low-income, and middle-income families, the students can identify, in a visual form, the percentage of the budget spent for the Basic 4. (Economic factor.)

2. As a small group project, the students can compile a list of foods eaten by their younger brothers and sisters, themselves, and their parents in social situations out of the home for a one-week period. (Social factor.)

3. Students individually may list their five favorite foods and their five least-liked foods. (Personal factor.)

4. When given the data provided by objectives 1, 2, and 3, the students in small group discussions can verbally assess the part an individual's financial situation, his social relationships, and his own personal tastes play in food-selection patterns.

From these examples the preprofessional should be able to discern the relationship of the specific behavioral objectives to the general objective and recognize that they are designed within the cognitive domain of learning. He will also note that there is a progression of learning taking place in the objectives. The first three provide the data which are necessary for the making of any analysis. In turn all meet the criteria for specific behavioral objectives stated earlier in the chapter.

The affective domain, as stated earlier, includes those objectives which involve interests, attitudes, emotions, values, or appreciations. In other words, the individual's "feelings" are the focal points in this domain.

Objectives in the affective domain direct the facilitator to provide for his students opportunities to explore their attitudes, take tentative positions, compare their logic with that of others, and revise their value systems.

Applying the criteria previously stated for specific behavioral objectives, the facilitator can generate meaningful objectives in the affective domain.

Assume that the same general objective is being utilized:

(The student is able) to analyze the factors which affect food-selection patterns.

Again a series of specific objectives can be planned which will provide data concerning present student values as reflected in their behavior:

1. When given the week's menus for the school cafeteria:
    a. Each student is able to list his choice for each day and give one written reason for each selection.
    b. Each student who would avoid eating at the school cafeteria on any given day is able to substitute
        1) where he would eat instead of the cafeteria;
        2) the foods he would eat; and
        3) one written reason for each choice.
2. From the list of reasons generated by the first objective for food selection, the students, through class discussion, are able to rank in order the five most important factors.
3. In small group discussions, the students are able to verbally analyze and record the effect that one of the five ranked factors had on their selection of food in relation to the nutritive value of the food selected.
    a. Group No. 1—Analyze the factor which was rank-ordered number five.
    b. Group No. 2—Analyze the factor which was rank-ordered number four.
    c. Group No. 3—Analyze the factor which was rank-ordered number three.
    d. Group No. 4—Analyze the factor which was rank-ordered number two.
    e. Group No. 5—Analyze the factor which was rank-ordered number one.

Each of the objectives is related to the general objective and meets the other criteria for specific behavioral objectives.

This series of objectives is potentially meaningful to high school students. One's choices of foods tend to be based on personal likes and dislikes without consideration being given to nutritive values. Thus by analyzing present behavior, the learners are forced to examine their own rationale. They then have the opportunity either to have their values reinforced or to reconsider their values in the light of the possible consequences.

Behavioral objectives that could be classified in the psychomotor domain will be fewer in number. As previously mentioned, the psychomotor domain focuses on some manipulative skill requiring neuromuscular coordination. In health education, opportunities to provide experiences of this nature are more limited, but they do exist. Again, using the same general objective,

(The student is able) to analyze the factors which affect food-selection patterns, one can devise behavioral objectives in the psychomotor domain that utilize learning activities pursued in the cognitive and affective domains.

1. In small groups the students are able to devise and act out a skit demonstrating situations in which their food-selection patterns are influenced by their finances, peer relationships, or their likes and dislikes.

2. The students in each of the five discussion groups are able to prepare a visual aid which shows

   a. the factor being analyzed,
   b. the types of foods students select,
   c. the nutritive value of the selected foods,
   d. the nutritive elements which are missing.

The skills developed in the above objectives are not of prime importance. The intent of objectives such as these is to actively involve students in their own learning. In addition, these objectives serve as a technique of feedback from the small groups to the total class. In this way, the class has the opportunity to hear, react to, and evaluate the analyses of all the groups.

The behaviorally stated objectives emphasized in this chapter are a key to improved instructional procedures. Look over the examples given once again. You will see that by identifying the behaviors, the facilitator has guidelines to follow, both in designing the learning experiences and in devising testing and evaluative procedures.

Table 2 provides some of the general action-words that may assist the neophyte in structuring behavioral objectives. Until these verbs are qualified by citing the specific behavior to be exhibited, one does not have a specific behavioral objective. Level 1 refers to early elementary, Level 2 to upper elementary, Level 3 to junior high, and Level 4 to high school. The designation of these terms at the various levels should not be construed as meaning they are never appropriate at other levels. The individual facilitator must determine for himself whether his students are capable of dealing with an abstract term. Of course, the ways in which the verbs are qualified will also be important.

In taking the big step forward toward improving learning effectiveness, the facilitator must understand the relationship of evaluation to behavioral objectives. Some exponents of behavioral objectives insist that a quantitative degree in evaluation must be attained. This is logical when the cognitive domain of learning receives the primary emphasis, as it does in some disciplines. In health education, however, to insist on quantification is illogical because the concepts do not lend themselves to *quantitative* evaluation as much as they do to *qualitative*.

TABLE 2

INFINITIVES USEFUL IN CONSTRUCTING GENERAL BEHAVIORAL OBJECTIVES

INFINITIVES	LEVEL 1	LEVEL 2	LEVEL 3	LEVEL 4
The student is able:				
To identify	X	X	X	X
To describe	X	X	X	X
To name	X	X	X	X
To point to	X	X	X	X
To compare	X	X	X	X
To cite	X	X	X	X
To construct		X	X	X
To order		X	X	X
To demonstrate		X	X	X
To develop		X	X	X
To examine		X	X	X
To contrast		X	X	X
To perform		X	X	X
To illustrate			X	X
To apply			X	X
To differentiate			X	X
To solve			X	X
To discriminate			X	X
To formulate				X
To integrate				X
To summarize				X
To interpret				X
To analyze	As Competencies Develop	As Competencies Develop	As Competencies Develop	X
To translate				X
To evaluate				X
To extrapolate				X
To synthesize				X

Accountability does not necessarily mean that the student must achieve a numerical competency level, but rather that he will be able to see possibilities for change in or reinforcement of his present health behaviors. The authors are not so much interested in forcing the student to regurgitate facts as they are in providing him with opportunities to express thoughts and feelings (affective domain) which he can match with those of his fellows. Evaluation of this kind of learning is possible and is demonstrated in chapter 8.

BREAKTHROUGH TOWARD CREATIVITY

Today's students are becoming increasingly disenchanted with their educational experiences. They aren't the first to have these feelings, but they are more vocal in expressing their frustration. It is a common occurrence to read news articles or hear television reports about student groups challenging existing requirements. How many of these comments are familiar?

- —"We have no identity. We're treated like a herd of cattle—go here—do this—don't do that."
- —"If my hair is clean and neat, why should I be suspended just because it's longer than the principal likes it?"
- —"Why can't I wear a pants suit to school when my mother can wear one to work and to parties?"
- —"What does what I wear and the length of my hair have to do with education anyway?"
- —"I'm putting in my time until I can quit. I'm not learning anything in school that has meaning for my life."
- —"Student Council is supposed to represent us. In reality, it's just the voice of the principal and the faculty."
- —"Students have no power unless they band together. When the blacks demonstrated, the administration got all up tight and made changes. Looks like the only way we can get change is to organize and demonstrate."
- —"That drug film was a bunch of crap. It gave the idea that some freak traps you into trying 'grass.' Man, my old man gave me my first 'joint.'"

No attempt will be made here either to analyze these comments or to put them in perspective. It is sufficient to observe that they are indicative of student frustration with existing educational practices, and of unrest; and represent a fervent plea for change.

Must change in teaching procedures be forced on the health educator by demonstration and confrontation? Has today's preprofessional forgotten his own dissatisfaction?

From a facilitator's standpoint, what changes are desirable and possible that may improve the instructional climate?

Providing opportunities wherein the students can be actively involved in their own learning is of prime importance. With the influx of more teachers oriented in the "facilitative model," the days of "I talk—you listen and learn" are numbered. The passive learner tends to be the bored, uninterested student. The uninterested student is often the disruptive one.

Generating Learning Experiences

The creation of meaningful learning experiences is influenced by the factors discussed in earlier chapters, namely: (1) knowledge about the particular students, (2) concepts pertinent to students, (3) major health problems in the school and community, (4) facilities, equipment, and resources available, (5) behavioral objectives constructed, and (6) content stated or implied in the objectives. The facilitator now has the basic information necessary to develop learning experiences that challenge students to be involved.

Unless the inexperienced teacher is part of a team, he is usually on his own in the initial planning. Thereafter students can contribute greatly toward evaluating the experiences. They will suggest modifications, eliminations, or additions to the available options. Avoid assuming that students lack ideas and creativity. Students are now more than ever recognized as one of education's greatest untapped resources.

How does the inexperienced preprofessional develop his competency to formulate significant experiences? It is obvious that he will lack much of the specific information it is desirable to have in planning for a specific group of students.

Resource Units. One device that has been found to be useful is the development of resource units. In college methods classes, small groups choose one of the concepts from the School Health Education Study (referred to at length in chapter 3) and determine the grade level in which they are interested. They then generate their own general behavioral objectives in all three domains and outline the content necessary for students to accomplish the objectives. The objectives also provide clues as to what types of learning experiences can be used.

These learning experiences provide students with opportunities to develop the capabilities stated in the objectives. To generate the greatest quantity of these experiences, most groups choose to brainstorm. During this process no evaluation is made of the suggestions.

After all the ideas are produced, each is evaluated on the basis of the following:

1. How will this activity assist students in exhibiting the stated behavior?
2. Does this experience actively involve the students?
3. Does this activity provide opportunities for students to express their individuality?
4. Does this activity provide opportunities for students to use their creativity?

The proposed learning experiences are then classified according to type: small group discussion, class discussion, debate, skit, survey, interview, computer-assisted instruction, learning-center activity, individual projects, value games.

Following this phase, the groups usually revert to working individually for the compilation of the most current, potentially useful teaching aids and references. See page 162 for a sample guide sheet. Each group's resource unit is then duplicated for every person in the class. Thus every individual has a personal file of six or seven resource units. These units serve several purposes. Each student has had the experience of helping to plan and to develop a unit. Each group has had to use its own ideas. All groups have had to become acquainted with a variety of sources to compile their finished products. In addition, each person has one or more units that he can utilize when he has an actual class. He need only change the behavioral objectives from general to specific. From the wide assortment of suggested learning experiences, he can select a variety which he thinks are relevant to his class. With these options, students have choices or an opportunity to suggest additions.

Student Involvement

As stated earlier, student involvement is essential for the most meaningful learning to occur. The facilitator's only limitation in planning these experiences is his own creativity. Financial outlay need rarely be a consideration. The remainder of this chapter gives some suggested learning experiences that may stimulate the production of other activities or modifications which can be utilized for a particular class.

Values and Games Students Play

Today's technology is bombarding students with a myriad of stimuli. They are removed from the comfortable, secure cocoon of the close-knit family, the parochial value system, and the local community mores that were experienced by past generations of students.

Consider the complexity of living in today's world. Television brings instant happenings from the campuses across the country. Today young people see film clips of yesterday's action in the Middle East and Far East conflicts. The Dow Jones average and gross national product (GNP) are common household terms. Space exploration has become so common that the names of the most current astronauts are almost unknown. The assassinations and funerals of world leaders are brought into the classrooms and homes live and in color.

The population is more mobile. Fathers are transferred to other cities, other states, or other countries. Fewer students remain in one community for the period of their entire school life. Thus forced changes are made in patterns of friendship.

The family unit is less stable. Both parents frequently work. School, church, and community have many organized activities that remove youth from the family influence. More homes are broken by divorce or death.

Is it any wonder that students have difficulty sorting out what is good or bad, what is reasonable or unreasonable, what is acceptable or unacceptable, what is appropriate or inappropriate? What opportunities are provided for them to develop their own value systems?

Unless students have opportunities to evaluate alternatives, how can they be expected to bring order out of confusion and make the judgments that are desirable for them?

A value system is made up of the elements important to an individual that provide guidelines for directing his life. It cannot be imposed successfully by either parents or teachers. The rejection by many of today's youth of the values cherished by their parents and/or teachers is quite evident.

To develop a system of values, one must go through a decision-making process. A value must be freely chosen; the alternatives with their resulting consequences must be evaluated; a decision must be made; and that decision *must be implemented*. This does not imply that a value is chosen for all time. Developing a value system is an ongoing process which may be modified or reinforced by experience, by feedback from others, by changing attitudes, or by new facts.

Game Strategies. Games can be of potential value as a seeding device to evoke later in-depth discussion and evaluation of alternatives.

Raths, Harmin and Simon suggest twenty-one teaching strategies that can be adapted to any subject matter field.[1] The following we have found to be very effective in introducing the affective areas pertaining to health education.

Values Voting is an informal poll made to determine where students stand. There are no teacher-imposed sanctions, nor is there any teacher-controlled

1. Louis E. Raths, Merrill Harmin, and Sidney Simon, *Values and Teaching* (Columbus, Ohio: Charles E. Merrill Co., 1966).

behavior, or manipulated choices. A series of phrases, statements, or questions is devised. At first these are teacher-developed. After becoming familiar with the technique, students develop lists that tend to be more relevant.

If the student is positive or agrees, he raises his hand; negative or disagrees, he turns thumb down; very positive, waves hand; very negative, stirs thumb; chooses not to vote, folds arms.

Below are several examples of how values-voting can be implemented in health education.

Friendship (agree-disagree)

1. It's uncomfortable to socialize with people you don't know.
2. It's more enjoyable to be with others than by yourself.
3. It's important to understand others' points of view.
4. When you have a personal problem, it's easier to talk it over with a friend than with parents.
5. Parents are more helpful than friends when you have a personal problem.
6. It's very important to have a "best" friend.
7. It's more important to have several good friends than to have a best friend.
8. Being a best friend involves a responsibility to that friend.
9. It's difficult for new students to develop friendships in this school.

Emotional Health (agree-disagree)

1. It's difficult to get along with people.
2. My parents don't understand me.
3. I often feel inadequate.
4. I eagerly look forward to what each day will bring.
5. I'm putting in time until I can quit school.
6. Teachers seem to have it in for me.
7. I look forward to weekends and vacations.
8. I enjoy life.

Fads (like-dislike). (Voting on both columns can be done by members of either or both sexes, or voting on either column can be done by members of the same or the opposite sex.)

Boys	*Girls*
1. Long sideburns	1. Maxi skirts
2. Moustaches	2. Mini skirts
3. Beards	3. Micro-mini skirts
4. Wigs	4. Wigs
5. Shoulder-length hair	5. Shoulder-length hair
6. Collar-length hair	6. Collar-length hair

Boys		*Girls*	
7.	Short hair	7.	Short hair
8.	Flairs	8.	Bell bottoms
9.	Bright-colored shirts	9.	Granny glasses
10.	Manti-hose	10.	Hot pants

We would suggest that no formal tally be made the first few times this technique is used. Until a facilitator has developed a rapport with his class and there is a climate of trust, students hesitate to risk expressing their true feelings.

Rank Ordering is a preference scale on which individual students rearrange a list of items.

Health Practices—Rank from most harmful to a person's health to least harmful.

A. 1. One marijuana cigarette per day.
    2. One alcoholic drink per day.
    3. One package of cigarettes per day.
    4. Never walking when it's possible to ride.
B. 1. Three marijuana cigarettes per day.
    2. Three alcoholic drinks per day.
    3. Three packages of cigarettes per day.
    4. Never walking when it's possible to ride.

Cultural Patterns and Food Choices—Rank from most liked to least liked.

1. Lasagna
2. Hamburger
3. Snails
4. Chitlins
5. Grits
6. Squid
7. Kielbasa

Health Practices—Rank items from most important long-term effect on personal health to least important.

1. Wash hands before eating.
2. Have yearly medical examination.
3. Periodic dental check-up.
4. Brush teeth after each meal.
5. Eat balanced meals.

Values Continuum is a method of generating the possible alternatives between two extremes. It is particularly useful for controversial areas —e.g., premarital sexual behavior, abortion, or use of contraceptives.

Premarital Sexual Experiences

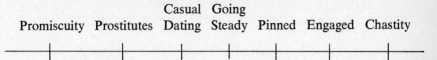

Casual Going
Promiscuity Prostitutes Dating Steady Pinned Engaged Chastity

When all the possible alternatives have been placed on the continuum, it can be used as a starting point for in-depth discussion of these questions in small groups or total class:

1. What are the possible consequences of each position on the continuum for girls? for boys?
2. What makes the various positions acceptable/unacceptable to you?
3. What behavior would be acceptable to you for your brother? your sister? your girlfriend? boyfriend?
4. What evidence do you have that the double standard still exists?
5. How do you decide what is right for you?

What are the alternative positions possible on this continuum?

Abortion

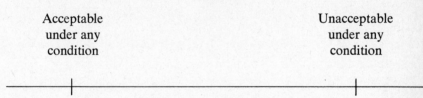

Acceptable
under any
condition

Unacceptable
under any
condition

Less sensitive areas also lend themselves to this technique. Personal positions can be plotted between the two extremes on such subjects as the frequency of wearing seat belts or the legalization of marijuana. In these cases the middle of the continuum can be reserved for the compulsive moderate who doesn't wish to commit himself.

As a follow-up, students on one side of the continuum may wish to talk with those on the other side. This is also a "natural" in identifying opposing views which can be tapped for the next game.

Table Talk is a method that calls for students holding opposing viewpoints to sit on opposite sides of a table. They discuss the rationale for their personal position for ten or fifteen minutes. Then they shift to the opposing viewpoint and try to support it. Since this often results in a pooling of ignorance due to lack of facts, references need to be available to enable students to find data that reflect or support the various positions.

We wish to reiterate that values are very personal in nature. They must be freely chosen and of sufficient importance to invite personal commitment.

The facilitator needs to remember that his personal value system may differ greatly from the systems presently held by his students. To be most effective he keeps lines of communication open. He neither rewards nor penalizes a student for accepting or rejecting his values. He makes a concerted effort to understand how things appear from the student's viewpoint. He avoids moralizing. He shares his own position, if asked, but does not try to impose it on others.

The inexperienced teacher need not hesitate to experiment with games. If one feels a little apprehensive, begin in a noncontroversial area. Modify one of the examples or develop one applicable to the class for which it is to be used. Risk! The resultant interaction will be a source of great satisfaction.

Crusade with Caution

The idealistic preprofessional may plunge into his teaching career with an evangelistic heart. He forsees the innumerable opportunities to help his students become well-adjusted, knowledgeable, healthier individuals. His philosophy may include total honesty in dealing with every issue in health education. In his own mind he may well be able to justify his position completely. Without meaning to stifle these commendable qualities, a warning signal must be hoisted before the facilitator falls into a trap of his own creation.

There are Controversial Areas in the Teaching of Health Education. Many individuals and groups in society are sensitive to schools teaching anything about reproduction, sexuality, dating, birth control, abortion, sexual deviate behavior, and even the venereal diseases. The facilitator must recognize that parents have rights to their beliefs, even though these may be in conflict with his own. He must avoid making the assumption that even though the health education program in his school has successfully included some of these subjects in the past, there is total acceptance by all. To assume this could be likened to sitting on a time bomb. When it explodes, the ramifications can be traumatic to the students, other parents, the teachers, the administration, the school, the school system, and the community. The facilitator must take precautions to defuse the bomb before it inflicts its destruction. What possible steps might he take?

He should examine the policies of the school and of the school system concerning teaching in these areas. If none exists, perhaps he might instigate moves to establish written guidelines. It is politic to involve parents and representatives of community groups in this endeavor.

The facilitator may choose to send a letter to all parents at the beginning of each school year describing what is to be learned, how it is going to be accomplished, and how the learning will be evaluated. Two other important items may be included in this letter:

1. An invitation to parents to visit the class at any time or call when questions arise;
2. An option for parents to have their children excluded from learning in an area that is in conflict with their beliefs. This arrangement can be made in advance in order that no undue social stigma may be inflicted upon the student and so that subtitute learning may be provided.

The facilitator may also consider the possibility of having a meeting with parents at the beginning of each semester so that they may examine the materials being used. Included may be the learning objectives, films, filmstrips, transparencies, and other resource materials. This idea is sound in that it can also provide an entree for parents to initiate discussions with their children in the home setting.

Providing a standardized form on which parents can submit in writing any objections they may have to what is being learned, the method employed, or the materials used may serve as a deterrent to a major upheaval. An example of this form will be found in Table 3. A suitable form can be designed to meet individual needs.

The facilitator should use the PTA, school newsletters, or even the local churches as vehicles for disseminating information about his program. Such dissemination is an excellent means of assuring the building of better public relations.

Although worksheets may be a valuable technique to use in some areas of learning, their use should be avoided when dealing with controversial issues. The less set down on paper the better, for without understanding the pre- or post-learning that takes place, someone may easily misinterpret words taken out of the larger context.

Nor is it always the new teacher who falls victim to conflicting philosophies. Very often the experienced facilitator develops a false sense of security. He may feel that because he has built his program over the years, with little or no objection having been raised, it couldn't happen to him. Ample documentation can be produced to show that such an explosion can and will occur.

The health educator sincerely believes that what he is offering to his students is valid and necessary. In order to protect himself and his program, he must accept and provide for differing philosophies. Thus he will be able to educate the majority of the students, those whose views are not opposed to such instruction. "Caution" is the key word in making plans for learning in possible problem areas.

TABLE 3

CITIZEN'S APPEAL CONCERNING THE TEACHING OF A CONTROVERSIAL ISSUE

Name ....

Address ....-...

Phone ....

I represent: ....myself

.................................organization. Name.................................

.................................group. Identify.................................

1. School in which incident or material was used?
   School ....
   Class ....
   Teacher involved ....
   Subject area ....
   Date of use ....

2. Statement of the problem? (please detail)

3. To what do you specifically object?

4. How did you obtain your information?
   ....your child (or children)
   ....your own observation
   ....reading reports, books, or seeing material
   ....hearing comments from other students
   ....hearing comments from other parents
   others: state ....

5. What action would you recommend?

6. Are you willing to attend a conference at school to discuss this matter?
   ....Yes
   ....No
   If yes, what times and days are best for your convenience?

   ....
   Signature
   ....
   Date

Citizen's Appeal Concerning the Teaching of a Controversial Issue (Courtesy Berea (Ohio) City School District)

The IMC and Health Education

Elementary and secondary schools that have committed themselves to breaking away from traditional incarceration recognize the student's need to have independent study time and facilities. Many have created instructional materials centers (IMC) where a learner may choose to go during his unassigned time or even during his class time if he is so directed by the teacher. These centers may be called by any one of numerous names, such as learning center, instructional resource center, educational materials center, media center, educational communication center, or, the term which will be here employed, instructional materials center (IMC). The uses to which such a center is put and the physical set-up in each individual school are as diversified as the labels given to it. Both are dependent upon the philosophy of the school itself and the imagination of the staff members.

In essence, the IMC is a combination library and audio-visual facility, usually manned by qualified paraprofessionals (aides). What is inside the IMC? Possibly all or some of the following:

Visual—Books, magazines, pamphlets, newspapers, clippings, slides, pictures, charts, maps, globes, felt kits.
Audio—Discs, cassette tapes, reel-to-reel tapes.
Audio-Visual—Films, filmstrips, television.
Tactile—Models, sculpture, globes, relief maps, building kits, games.
Equipment—Record players, tape recorders, radios, a central sound system, portable public-address system, cameras, television receivers, video tape recorders, motion-picture projectors, teaching machines, filmstrip viewers and projectors, opaque and overhead projectors, projection screen, photocopy equipment, slide projectors, slide viewers, dry mount presses, and a computer terminal.

The IMC can be an invaluable supplement to the health education program. Students may choose to:

1. Browse or satisfy personal health educational interests;
2. Teach one another (nobody teaches children better than children);
3. Make up work missed because of absence;
4. Pursue individual or group projects/reports;
5. Utilize electronic learning devices to increase the depth of their understanding;
6. Work with models or devise their own learning aids;
7. Prepare student-structured classroom presentations;
8. Work on continuous learning tasks as prescribed by the facilitator; or
9. Partake of evaluative activities to measure their achievement level.

Besides providing independent-learning opportunities for the student, the IMC, on occasion, allows the facilitator the chance to work with fewer numbers in the classroom. Thus more individual attention is possible.

The paraprofessionals in the IMC help the learner to help himself with the materials and equipment available. If the health education facilitator provides the aides with copies of his concept plan, including behavioral objectives, learning activities, and evaluative procedures, they will be better able to give the student meaningful help. Also the student will be able to take care of remedial obligations. In addition the facilitator must provide the IMC with the necessary filmstrips, tapes, films, references, and other instructional materials necessary to implement the specific learning objectives.

Where the schools, many of which have not as yet reached this level of development, do not provide the student with the opportunities available in an IMC, the health educator should not be dismayed. Rather he must recognize immediately another challenge to his ingenuity. Why not create a health-education learning center within his own room? It doesn't need to be elaborate. The facilitator can start with a corner of the room or with even an unused storage room. For a beginning he needs only the basic necessities such as outlets, lighting, tables, wall space, and shelving. If available he may get a four-wheel cart on which to move the references borrowed from his own library or from some other library within his school system that is not dealing with the same concept at the same time.

Here are a few additional suggestions which may be followed in undertaking such a project:

1. *Start where you are now.* Begin building upon whatever you have in materials, classroom collections, audio-visual aids.
2. *Study materials and methods.* Collect information.
3. *Evaluate what you now have.*
4. *Determine goals.* Think in terms of the immediate interim, and long-range phases. What will be needed? Start thinking about space for viewing, listening, conferences, and individual study even if it is in small corners of the room.
5. *Build slowly and carefully.* List all materials (books, films, filmstrips, models, charts, posters, etc.) in your own catalog and keep it up to date.
6. *Keep flexible. Keep current. Keep looking ahead.* Goals may change as new ideas develop. New materials and teaching methods will be produced and developed.
7. Invite the students to use the room at any time they can even though a class may be in session. Who knows—you may motivate those who make decisions to establish an IMC for the total school.

Continuous Progress Learning

"Student involvement" in his own learning is certainly one of the key phrases in the philosophy of this book. One of the more potentially successful means of getting learners actively involved is the continuous-progress method of learning in a given health concept. Continuous-progress learning (CPL) means that the facilitator plans individualized activities to be undertaken by the learner based upon the behavioral objectives and the learning ability of his students. These learning tasks are then undertaken

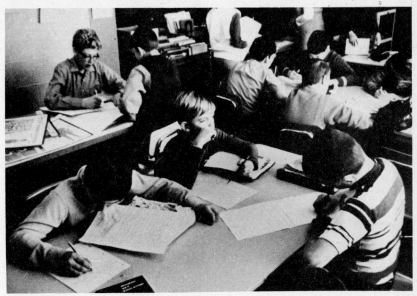

— Photo by Steven Goldman

Continuous Progress Learning

and accomplished by the student at his own rate of speed, working individually or in groups of two or more.

How may a continuous-learning program be set by the facilitator? The health concept may be divided into several parts based upon the general behavioral objectives. Each part will have specific behavioral objectives, from which the facilitator will draw the individualized activities to be prescribed. Copies of the specific objectives and the student learning tasks can be posted or given to the learner as a guide sheet.

There are innumerable types of activities that the learner may use to reach a specific objective. He may view filmstrips, listen to tape recordings, study transparencies, work with models, evaluate movies, complete guide sheets using books, pamphlets, or periodicals, carry out experiments, interact in small group discussions on objective-related topics of the group's choice, conduct original surveys, or, if available, partake of computer-assisted instruction. When the learner completes the activities, he is then evaluated to see whether the learning objective has been reached. If the degree of competency desired is achieved, he then moves on to the next part; and thus he progresses continuously.

It should be noted that certain guidelines need to be considered before undertaking a continuous-progress learning program in health education:

1. Does the concept lend itself well to CPL?

2. Are the learners involved concurrently in CPL in other disciplines?
3. Are sufficient resources available?

If the answers to items 1 and 3 are yes, and if the student is not being bombarded by CPL in many areas of his learning experience, then the facilitator may find this is a very valuable avenue of pursuit. CPL may prove to be very gratifying to both the learner and the facilitator for many reasons:

1. A relaxed atmosphere in the classrooms prevails.
2. There is a more personalized relationship between the learner and the facilitator (informal give and take).
3. There is the possibility for reciprocal learning (peer tutoring) with discoveries and/or value judgments shared.
4. It is possible to have individualized objectives tailored to the learning abilities of the student.
5. The slow, average, or fast learner has complete freedom to work at his own level or speed without handicapping or conflicting with the others.
6. Individualized guidance is possible.
7. The student and the facilitator can observe the activity and the performance in relation to the objective.
8. CPL represents a "change of pace" in method from the regular classroom process.
9. The student is actively involved in his learning.

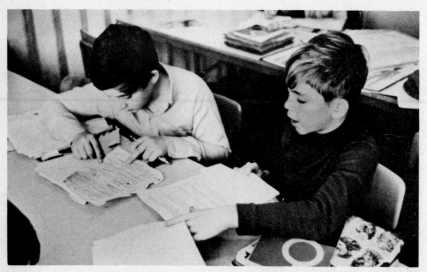

— Photo by Steven Goldman

Continuous Progress Learning

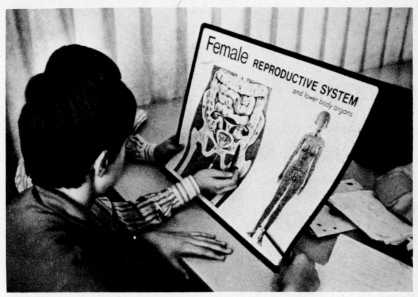

— Photo by Steven Goldman

Continuous Progress Learning

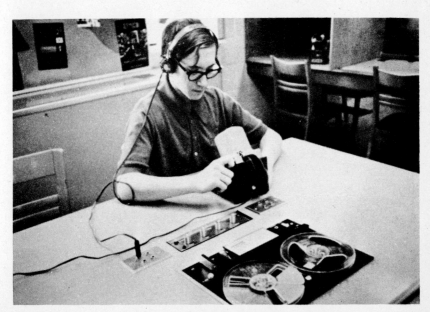

— Photo by Steven Goldman

Instructional Materials Center

10. Eventual success is within the grasp of every student, whatever his ability. With help from the facilitator and his peers there is little fear of failure.
11. The learner may possibly evaluate his own work so that he can recognize his weak points.

On the other hand, the facilitator must be aware of some of the additional responsibilities required to insure success if he chooses to undertake CPL.

1. The facilitator must be able to recognize the learning ability levels of his students.
2. It is very time-consuming to preplan and to evaluate progress.
3. Much office time and help are necessary for duplicating materials.
4. The role of the facilitator within the classroom is just that—"facilitator." He must be able to refer the learner to the necessary resources to perform his learning tasks.
5. A variety of reference materials and learning aids must be available to the learner.
6. Imagination on the part of the facilitator is a requisite in designing tasks that are interesting, relevant, and meaningful.
7. It would be advisable not to undertake CPL at the beginning of the school year. Since there is a close relationship between the facilitator and the learner in this learning method, there must be time for this rapport and trust to develop.

Another interesting ramification of CPL that the facilitator may consider using is the "open classroom." This means encouraging the student to come to the health education room during his study halls or any other unassigned time to use the resources and continue to work on his learning activities. He may enter regardless of whether there is a class in session or not. If the facilities seem to shrink, the facilitator will just have to move in more folding chairs. And if interest is really generated (and it may well be), the facilitator may even find himself eating his lunch in the room in order to be available to his students. What great opportunities are available for individualized guidance to take place! Such rewards to both the learner and the facilitator!

To summarize, it should be pointed out that for continuous-progress learning to be effective, the learner and the facilitator have responsibilities:

Facilitator	*Learner*
1. To choose a concept that lends itself well to CPL.	1. Be aware of the objectives to be reached.

2. To consider the needs and abilities of his students and devise effective general and specific behavioral objectives.

2. Carry out the behavioral activity with understanding.

3. To designate imaginative learning activities to reach the objectives.

3. Cooperate in the evaluation procedures.

4. To use many evaluative methods.

Continuous-progress learning is a school experience that offers the learner the opportunity to develop as an individual human being according to his abilities. The preprofessional health educator should strongly consider employing CPL at some time during the school year.

The Computer in Health Education

No longer must one gaze into a crystal ball to foresee the day when computers will be an integral part of learning. Computer-programmed learning is now a reality in many schools in many areas. Perhaps the only need one might have for the crystal ball now would be to look into the future and see oneself in the picture as a designer of learning experiences.

Almost inevitably computerized instruction will become a valuable part of the American educational system, which is already deeply involved with data processing (report cards, student records, payroll, attendance, scheduling, inventory, etc.).

The preprofessional must not be misled by this revolution in learning method—the computer does not pretend to be replacing the health education facilitator. Instead, it offers him another method of supplementing his teaching effectiveness and challenges his creativity to make learning more individualized, relevant, and interesting to his students. Its utilization as a direct individualized learning device *frees the facilitator*—enables him to aid his students on a personal one-to-one basis and not be bogged down in monitorial duties. Neither should the computer be thought of as a method for testing. In keeping with the philosophy of this book, the teacher's role becomes one of *facilitating* the specific learning of students and not mass dosing them in the traditional manner as if learners were not variable.

There are two types of computerized programs that lend themselves well to health education and with which preprofessionals should be acquainted. These are Computer-Assisted Instruction (CAI) and Computer-Managed Instruction (CMI).

Computer-Assisted Instruction. Computer-assisted instruction (CAI) is defined as instruction (in addition to normal classroom activity) using a computer terminal. Schools with philosophies that include offering the student every opportunity to participate in the management of his own education are either now using CAI or are moving in this direction.

Many schools are using time-sharing CAI in cooperation with another school to alleviate some of the cost problems. Some schools even have their own "in-house" systems. Students may use the computer individually (a) during free time, (b) as an activity in a continuous-progress learning program, (c) as a station in an instructional learning center, or (d) during class time as an assigned activity for personalized instruction. It is also possible to use one computer terminal for a small group of from two to four. Here the participants discuss the alternative selections given and decide on a group answer. One person enters the response on the typewriter terminal.

Schools that utilize team teaching are in an advantageous position in utilizing CAI. Part of the team can work directly with students and part can be writing instructional materials to be programmed. With some moderate instruction, the facilitator can generate questions or statements, in either the cognitive or affective domain, that correspond to the specific behavioral objectives. Coupled with these, he would design comments to reinforce the correctness or explain the incorrectness of answers selected

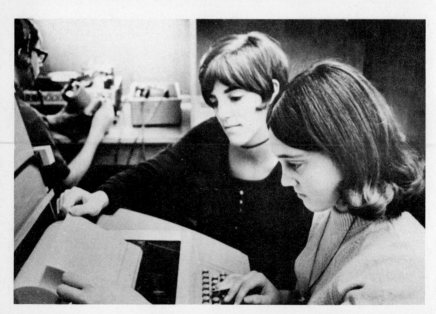

— Photo by Steven Goldman

Computer Assisted Instruction

by the learner in the cognitive domain, and offer judgmental alternatives in the affective domain. The lesson would then be converted into computer language by the programmer.

As the learner runs the program of tasks as written in the cognitive domain, he answers the questions set forth and immediately knows whether his answer is correct or incorrect. If he is wrong, he is told why he is wrong and is given the option of trying another answer. Programmed instruction in this domain is easily adapted to CAI and is all the more effective in that the student cannot see the answer until he has made his selection.

The following is an example of a computerized question in the cognitive domain:

Directions: Type in the *LETTER* of the choice that makes this statement most correct.

1. Self-medication over a period of time may:

		Computer Response
A.	Disguise symptoms of a serious nature.	Products containing aspirin may reduce the discomfort from pain to a level where one does not seek medical advice. Choice A is only a partial answer. Is there not a better answer? Try again.
B.	Encourage the spreading of a communicable disease.	The symptoms of some diseases will disappear whether or not they are treated. Self-medication if one has contracted syphillis would be dangerous because the chancre will disappear, but the disease is still present. Choice B is only a partial answer. Is there not a better answer? Try again.
C.	Aggravate existing conditions.	When we prescribe for our own symptoms, we run a risk that the medication we choose to take might be the worst thing for the actual condition. Thus the person who, thinking his abdominal cramps are from constipation, takes a laxative risks a burst appendix and peritonitis. Choice C is only a partial answer. Is there not a better answer? Try again.
D.	Result in A, B, and C.	You are correct. For additional information on each choice, type A; read the response, then type B; then C.

The most challenging problem to the health educator who has the computer terminal at his disposal is how to use it most effectively to assist his instruction. He needs to be aware that a CAI lesson is not limited to the cognitive domain or the simple recall of knowledge. Tasks involving the affective domain can also be implemented through CAI. An example of this would be:

1. Sex ....M ....F

2. Do you smoke? ....Yes ....No.

3.A-1   If your answer is *yes:*
Below are 6 factors that may influence a non-smoker to become a smoker. Inspect the list. Which influenced you?

    A.   Mother smokes
    B.   Father smokes
    C.   Close friends smoke
    D.   Improvement of self-image
    E.   Seeking attention
    F.   Rebelling against authority

3.A-2   *Directions.* Rank order by placing the *LETTERS* of the factors opposite the numbers in descending order from most important to the least important.

    1.............
    2.............
    3.............
    4.............
    5.............
    6.............

3.A-3   If the most important factor that influenced you to smoke is *NOT* in the above list type it here:

3.B-1   If your answer is *NO:*
Below are 7 factors which may influence a person *NOT* to smoke. Inspect the list. Which influenced you?

    A.   Cost of smoking
    B.   Non-acceptance by friends
    C.   Parental objections
    D.   Training rules
    E.   Objectionable taste
    F.   Objectionable odor
    G.   Surgeon-general's report

3.B-2   *Directions:* Rank order by placing the *LETTERS* of the factors
       opposite the numbers in descending order from most important to
       least important.

    1.............
    2.............
    3.............
    4.............
    5.............
    6.............
    7.............

3.B-3   If the most important factor that is influencing you not to smoke is
       NOT in the above list, type it here:

The results of such a study can then be tabulated by the computer and the
results assessed by the learners in a small group discussion.

The possibility of utilizing the psychomotor domain in CAI is not
inconceivable. It was mentioned previously in this chapter that students
are one of the greatest untapped resources of learning. If the school has
the use of a computer, it is likely that some of the students are learning
simple programming techniques in their mathematics class. Perhaps their
talents and imagination might be employed in developing student-designed
computerized programs in health education geared to the behavioral objectives in a given concept. Interdisciplinary learning is relevant learning.

If a computer is available in a school, CAI is limited only by the creativity of the health educator. Have you heard this before? The facilitator
can plan instructional lessons to (1) enhance student learning, (2) present
options not previously considered, and (3) reinforce present knowledge.

There are probably two outstanding disadvantages that must be cited
in the use of CAI. One is that limited school funds may inhibit its utilization. The other is that CAI is limited to one person per terminal. Since this
is so, the facilitator may find an even more cost-effective use of the computer just as exciting. Computer-Managed Instruction (CMI) is a possible
alternative.

Computer-Managed Instruction. In this method the computer is used
to monitor and record student progress and make assignments according
to areas of weakness. A typical sct-up is the following:

1. Learners take a preliminary diagnostic test (pretest) from which the
   computer scores results and records areas of weakness.
2. On the basis of this the computer gives the student an assignment
   (i.e., continuous-progress unit) that is appropriate to his weakness.
3. The learner completes test answers at the end of the unit on a card
   which the computer scores and records and then issues the next assignment dependent upon the learner's progress.

Initiating this approach is extremely time-consuming, but it completely frees the facilitator for activities other than record-keeping. In addition, the learning task is completely individualized.

The preprofessional health education facilitator must be aware of the trend toward this type of educational technology, and must open his mind to learning the techniques involved in preparing lessons that can be computerized.

Original Surveys

Another potentially useful learning experience is the student-developed survey. Within some broad concepts the local survey can provide students with the current base-line data against which to compare their own knowledge, practices, experiences, or opinions.

What criteria could the facilitator apply in considering the desirability of having students construct a survey instrument? The guidelines can be divided into those that are general and those that are specific.

The general criteria would apply toward the evaluation of any potential activity. Assuming that these were answered in the affirmative, then the criteria specific to surveys would be applied.

General:
1. Will the activity enable students to achieve any of the stated behavioral objectives?
2. Will the activity provide students with a more meaningful experience than any other activity?
3. Can the results be used in a way that will enhance the learning of the students?

Specific:
1. What population would it be valuable to survey?
2. With guidance, do these students have the ability to construct a useful instrument?
3. Will it be feasible for the students to administer the instrument?
4. Can the results be tabulated quickly?

There are many populations that could provide data on a variety of topics. Within the school, surveys could be developed that assess present or desired knowledge, present practices, present opinions, past experiences, or any combination. Any grade level or all grade levels represented in a school could be sampled.

Within the community, the population to be surveyed could be the students' parents, neighbors, representative individuals from local business and/or industry. Which population is used would depend upon the purpose of the survey. Table 4 suggests several ways in which surveys can be utilized, dependent upon the purpose for which they were designed.

TABLE 4

ORIGINAL SURVEYS

POPULATION	TYPE	PURPOSE	USE
Own Class	Desired knowledge	Interests	Grouping for future learning-center activity
	Present knowledge	Preassessment	Selection of learning experiences
Grade Level	Present practices	Comparison with own practices	Small group or class discussion—reasons for differences and similarities
Grade Level/ School/ Parents/ Neighbors	Present opinions	Comparison with own opinions	Basis for differences and similarities. Collection of reference materials to support various viewpoints.
Business/ Industry	Community problems	Identify local problems	Plan student involvement in community

As with all potential learning experiences, there are advantages as well as disadvantages in using original surveys. The facilitator will have to decide on the desirability of using the survey.

Advantages:

1. Students have to respond with some initial research in order to devise the statements or questions.
2. They have an opportunity to get the information that is of interest and value to them.
3. Development of the instrument provides an opportunity for cooperative action.
4. Administering the instrument provides an opportunity for student interaction with a variety of people.
5. Students can use their creativity in planning a unique method of presenting the results to the entire class.
6. It is an opportunity to plan, administer, present, and evaluate an original research project.
7. If well done, the instrument can be used for future classes.
8. It provides an opportunity for students to interpret the results within the framework of diverse responses.

Disadvantages:

1. It is time consuming to develop, to administer, and to apply the survey.
2. Administering the instrument can be disruptive of other classes.
3. It can be "busy work" if the application of the results is overshadowed by enthusiasm for the instrument.

When the facilitator decides that a survey would be of significant value, he must prepare himself to assist the students. Prior to the time the project is undertaken, he should arrange to have reference materials available for the groups of students. Information will be needed not only on the topic but also about survey procedures. Examples of various types of survey instruments are most useful in assisting students to choose the form and the type of responses that will suit their purpose.

Serving as a consultant to the planning group, the facilitator can raise thought-provoking questions. The intent here is to focus on procedure and content rather than to manipulate students to develop the instrument that the instructor wants.

Examples of this type of question would be:

1. Specifically, what do you want to find out?
2. From whom do you want this information?
3. What type of statement or question will enable you to get the desired information?

4. What information do you need about the topic?
5. Where can you find the information you need?
6. What type of scale or response will be the most valuable?
7. How practical is what you are planning?
8. How can the results be used?

When the instrument has been devised, it is desirable to administer it to a small number of people. This trial run enables the group to make revisions to improve the clarity of the statements before applying the survey on a full scale basis.

Following the administration and the tabulation of the instrument, the results can be utilized in a variety of ways. Commonly a group report of the findings is issued. This tends to be very sterile in that it tends to become the termination when, in fact, it should be only the beginning. If no use is to be made of the results beyond the report, one might question the value of the time spent.

The results may be programmed for the computer. Members of the entire class could then respond to the survey statements or questions. The resulting comparisons of practices or opinions could then become the basis for small group or class discussions.

Some type of discussion is vital for alerting students to the limitations inherent in the survey technique. When all students have been involved in some phase of the survey—developing, administering, tabulating, programming, or answering—the unmeasured variables become more meaningful to them.

Breaking out of the lock-step of traditionalism, as the preprofessional must have concluded by now, is not an easy matter. But if health education is to move forward and gain its rightful position in the lives and education of students, there must be facilitators who:

1. Are willing to try to innovate methods and procedures for best motivating student learning;
2. Do not believe that their education ends with their degree and
   a. actively participate in professional organizations,
   b. read professional writings,
   c. participate in in-service workshops,
   d. attend seminars and conferences, and
   e. make visitations to see how other health education departments function;
3. Will break through the self-imposed barriers to creativity and implement their ideas;
4. Will make health education relevant to the needs of today's youth.

A valid and consuming question that has perhaps "zinged" the preprofessional in reading this chapter is, "When do I get time for all this?"

Remember that one must build gradually. Bear in mind, also that many school systems offer their staff members the opportunity for remuneration during the summer months for writing materials such as have been described here. Usually this involves writing a proposal describing the activity the facilitator wishes to undertake, the need for the project, the objectives, and the procedures. School systems that offer this opportunity have guidelines for the proposal initiator to follow. The health education facilitator may wish to investigate such opportunities.

Summary

Creativity in teaching provides more satisfying interactions for both students and facilitators. The potential exists for both learning and teaching to be exciting as well as rewarding.

The learning experiences suggested in this chapter make use of the less traditional teaching methods as well as newer technological teaching aids. Facilitators can be equally creative in adapting the more traditional teaching methods. These will be discussed in the next chapter.

Begin now to develop materials for Values Games, for Continuous-Progress Learning Programs, for the Computer-Assisted Instruction, and to collect materials that will be useful in helping students develop original surveys.

BREAKING OUT OF THE LOCK STEP

In today's generation of socially aware college students lies the hope for implementing the desperately needed change in educational teaching methodology. Now is the time to break out of the lock step that has entrapped so many teachers of yesterday and today.

Why should educators feel obligated to teach the way they were taught? Is the image of what an educator is, what he does, and how he does it so sacrosanct that promoting change would shatter the foundation of education? Is the risk so great that he dare not try?

There is really nothing sacred about teaching methods. What are the reasons so many teachers continue to utilize the traditional methods in traditional ways? Perhaps they have read the methods texts extolling the virtues of the traditional methods. Perhaps they have been in methods classes where innovative methods were discussed but not experienced. Perhaps they feel most comfortable in replicating the methods to which they themselves have been exposed. Whatever the reason, teachers who are interested in becoming facilitators of learning will resist being limited by traditionalism. This is not meant to imply that traditional methods have no place in the educational structure. Rather, the plea is being made for the facilitator to change his focus. That focus, instead of being upon what he (the teacher) wants to accomplish, should be on what competencies the students should be able to exhibit. This change of focus will lead the facilitator to search for the existing methods, a modification of an existing method, or the development of methods more effective in helping his students to achieve the desired competencies.

No method exists that can be labeled as "the" method to use to develop competency "x" or competency "y." Students are not computers that can be programmed in standard ways to secure standard results. Consequently the facilitator must constantly be searching for means that will challenge students to develop their own capabilities.

The next section will include a brief description of each teaching method, a chart listing the advantages and disadvantages of each method, and suggestions or modifications to increase the opportunities for student involvement.

Teaching Methods

Contract Method (Dalton Plan). This may be either an informal, unsigned contract or a formal, signed contract. It covers a designated period of time, usually the length of time spent on a concept, on a unit, or on a topic. Is consists of a series of three subcontracts, usually preplanned by the instructor. There is a minimum, or "C" contract that specifies the requirements all students must accomplish to receive a "C" grade. The second part, designated "B," designates additional requirements for a "B" grade. The third section gives more assignments which, if successfully completed, result in an "A" grade.

If an informal contract is used, the student works through the assignments, having them checked or evaluated, and completes as many as possible within the allotted time.

When a formal, signed contract is used, the student determines how much of the contract he wishes to do. He is then responsible for completing the amount for which he contracted. The stipulation is usually made that a contract may be renegotiated downward but not upward.

Contract Method

Advantages	*Disadvantages*
Teacher:	Teacher:
1. Can prepare contract before classes begin.	1. Spends excessive amount of time evaluating completed assignments.
2. Has time to assist individual students.	2. Must define standards for acceptable performance.
Student:	Student:
1. Is aware of the objectives to be reached.	1. Is pressured to fulfill contract.
2. Knows what has to be done.	2. May overestimate own ability.
3. Is forced to organize his time.	3. Unless motivated, can get by on minimum effort.
4. Works at own pace.	4. Can never do more than originally contracted for.
5. Knows where he stands at all times.	5. Must spend a great deal of time preparing material.
6. Who is more capable is given opportunity to excel.	6. Has little opportunity for interaction with other students.
7. Assumes responsibility for completing contract.	7. Can receive limited help from

8. Can renegotiate if circumstances warrant.
9. Becomes more familiar with outside resources.

General:
1. Reduces competition between students.
2. Reduces opportunities for subjective evaluation.
3. Increases objective evaluation.
4. Encourages students to be self-directing.

teacher on work done outside of class.
8. Has no opportunity to suggest activities meaningful to him.

General:
1. Pre-planned contract lacks flexibility.

The contract method can be modified. Modification makes the contracts more flexible, gives students an opportunity to influence activities, encourages them to use their initiative and creativity, makes possible the inclusion of activities meaningful to them, and reduces their chances of failure. Contracts offer opportunity for continuous learning. Modifications:

1. Open-ended contract "A." Each student is enabled to devise a project he is interested in pursuing.
2. Develop a series of three or four contracts tailored to differing abilities from which students can choose.
3. One contract with three or four options given for each subcontract.
4. Same as #3 above, with each subcontract having one or more spaces within which the student can devise his own project.

Student-developed projects must meet the following criteria:

1. They must be related to the concept for which the contract has been constructed.
2. They must aid the student in exhibiting the behavior designated in the behavioral objective.
3. Proposals must be written up and approved by the facilitator.

Debate Method. This consists of a formal presentation of the affirmative and negative sides of a topic by two teams. Each team consists of two people. Topics controversial in nature make the best debate topics. For example, note each of the following statements. (In any community, there would be adherents of opposing viewpoints. The topics are timely, and reference material to support either viewpoint would be readily available.)

Resolved: Existing antipollution laws should be rigorously enforced.
Resolved: The use of marijuana should be legalized.

Resolved: The sale of tobacco and tobacco products should be banned.
Resolved: Contraceptive information and devices should be available
to anyone regardless of age or marital status.

Limits on presentation time need to be adjusted depending on the
amount of time available. Since the purpose of this method differs from
that of competitive debate, rarely would more than half the available time
be used for the total presentation, to allow for follow-up procedures with
the remainder of the class. A suggested schedule for a 50-minute class
period would be:

Moderator—Introduction 2 min.
Affirmative #1—Presentation 5 min.
Negative #1—Presentation 5 min.
Negative #2—Rebuttal 5 min.
Affirmative #2—Rebuttal 5 min.
Negative #1—Concluding remarks 2 min.
Affirmative #1—Concluding remarks 2 min.
Follow-up Procedures—15 to 20 min.
Assignment and miscellaneous—4 to 9 min.

Debate Method

Advantages

Teacher:
1. Has basis for evaluation.
2. May obtain new information.
3. Can design follow-up procedures based on presentation.

Student:
1. Can develop his reasoning ability.
2. Is forced to organize his thoughts.
3. Has opportunity to speak to an audience.
4. Plans cooperatively with teammate.
5. Becomes familiar with divergent views through reference materials used.

Disadvantages

Teacher:
1. Must be knowledgeable about subject.
2. Needs to have a quantity of reference materials available.
3. Needs time to assist the teams during their preparation period.

Student:
1. If poorly prepared, handicaps his team.
2. Is at a disadvantage if he is afraid to speak before an audience.
3. Is under pressure to make his point within the time limit.

General:

1. Can be highly motivational for the bright student.

General:

1. Only a limited number of students can participate.
2. Controversial topic may be objectionable to community.
3. Solutions to problem are limited by the statements.

It would be unusual for a facilitator to have a class in which the majority of the students felt at ease speaking before the class. The formal debate can be modified to enable more students to be involved and to reduce the threat posed by a large audience for the timid student. Modifications:

1. Class divided into groups of ten to twelve seated in informal circles. Debate teams give presentations while seated. All teams are functioning simultaneously. Facilitator moves as unobtrusively as possible from group to group, gathering data to use in follow-up. Where team-teaching is used, each facilitator can be responsible for two or three groups.
2. When classes meet in small groups, the "Table Talk" idea (see p. 57) can be utilized. If the group is less than fifteen, the entire class can be divided into affirmative and negative teams. Individuals are given two minutes to present alternate sides.
3. To utilize the "Table Talk" idea with a group of more than fifteen, use teams of four or six. Nonparticipants are observers.

Demonstration Method. Normally the teacher has set up equipment that attempts to clarify some concept. For example, a beef heart may be dissected, various first-aid techniques may be shown, blood samples may be used to show hemoglobin content or blood-typing reactions. The demonstration is done by the teacher.

Demonstration Method

Advantages

Teacher:

1. Tends to capture student attention.
2. Can prepare material prior to class.
3. May motivate student interest.

Disadvantages

Teacher:

1. Needs skill to use equipment effectively.
2. May be embarrassed if demonstration fails.
3. Needs time to organize and set up the demonstration.
4. Requires equipment that may be expensive.

Advantages	*Disadvantages*

Student:
1. Gets a better understanding from a visual presentation.
2. Tends to retain more.
3. Tends to be interested and attentive.

General:
1. Effective for small groups.
2. Adds variety to class.

5. May create disciplinary problems if entire class can't see.
6. Is the only person who develops demonstrating skill.

Student:
1. Can miss meaning of demonstration.
2. May find it difficult to see.
3. Isn't personally involved in the demonstration.

General:
1. Time-consuming.
2. Student participation is negligible.
3. Difficult for all to see if used with large groups.

Alterations can be made to encourage students to develop their skills in demonstrating and clarifying. In addition, the problem of the students not being able to see the demonstration can be greatly reduced. Modifications:

1. A series of three or four demonstrations can be set up in different parts of the classroom. A student can be in charge of each station responsible for setting up the demonstration and explaining it to segments of the class as they move from station to station. The facilitator will need to work with the demonstrators prior to class. During the demonstrations he is freed to give assistance as needed.

2. If expensive equipment is not involved, several identical demonstrations can be given simultaneously using student demonstrators. The role of the facilitator is, again, that of assisting as needed. The class is divided so that all may be in close proximity to a demonstration.

Discussion Method. This is a commonly used method which encourages verbal interaction between students. To a lesser degree, there will be student-to-teacher interaction. When the facilitator is unskilled in involving students, discussions cease and the class tends to become a recitation or question-and-answer session.

Discussion Method

Advantages	Disadvantages
Teacher:	Teacher:
1. Can keep discussion "on track" without being the central figure.	1. Needs knowledge that goes beyond any textbook.
2. Can encourage students to express ideas and opinions.	2. Must be comfortable with an informal atmosphere.
3. Can encourage students to support their position with documented proof.	
Student:	Student:
1. Has opportunity to develop reflective thinking.	1. May lack sufficient knowledge to discuss topic.
2. Has an equal opportunity to participate.	2. May hesitate to participate if he is shy.
3. Can exchange ideas with others.	3. May dominate the discussion if he is aggressive.
4. Can express personal opinions.	
5. Becomes aware of divergent opinions.	
6. Has opportunity to evaluate diverse ideas.	
General:	General:
1. Enables students to share common problems.	1. Is time-consuming.
2. Misunderstandings can be clarified.	2. Getting sidetracked may occur repeatedly.
	3. May become a "pooling of ignorance."
	4. Tends to be overused.
	5. Large class limits discussion.

To use this method effectively, the facilitator needs to develop skills in involving students and in phrasing thought-provoking statements or questions. (Nothing kills a discussion more quickly than a question that can be answered by yes or no.) He also needs to resist using his status to dominate the discussion. Arranging the seating so that students may talk to each other face to face is helpful. It is difficult to carry on a discussion with someone's back. The arrangement by which everyone is seated in rows facing the teacher encourages all comments to be made to the teacher. With practice, the facilitator develops techniques to turn the discussion away from himself—e.g., "Who has evidence to support that statement/opinion?" or "If I understand you correctly, you were saying you are in favor of .... Under what conditions would this action be desirable/undesirable?"

Field Trips. Technically, any time a class is moved outside the normal classroom for purposes of enrichment, that move constitutes a field trip. Although only community resources are usually considered, one should not overlook various parts of the school itself as a learning laboratory. To be most effective, any field trip must be carefully planned, organized, and implemented. Only then will this method effectively supplement, enrich, and interpret classroom activities.

Field Trip Method

Advantages	*Disadvantages*
Teacher:	Teacher:
1. Receives assistance from person who is knowledgeable in field.	1. Must spend great deal of time in organizational and administrative detail.
2. Becomes more familiar with community resources.	2. May have difficulty evaluating outcomes.
3. Can provide a meaningful experience for his students.	3. Is responsible for health and safety of students.
4. Has opportunity to associate with students in a more informal atmosphere.	4. May have disciplinary problems.
Student:	Student:
1. Has opportunity to see actual process.	1. May miss other classes.
2. Has a change of scene and activity.	2. May not be able to afford the expense.
3. Can make observations in the real setting.	3. May be distracted by surroundings.
4. Will be better prepared to discuss experience.	4. Has difficulty taking notes.
5. Becomes aware of resources.	
6. Can have his interest aroused.	
7. Has opportunity to ask questions.	
8. Can see practical application of concepts discussed.	

General:

1. Can be very motivating.
2. Can be enjoyable as well as meaningful.
3. May provide stimulus for further study.

General:

1. Can be expensive.
2. Seeing and hearing can be a problem with a large group.
3. May not fulfill the purpose.
4. Other teachers may object.

Must all the planning for a field trip be done by the teacher? When given the opportunity, students gain valuable experience by having some of the responsibilities. Obviously this will take more time, but the results tend to make it worthwhile. When the facilitator assumes that students are capable and gives the guidance necessary, students are successful. Again we are advocating students becoming involved in their own learning. Start with elementary youngsters and the school with which they are familiar. With each experience they develop more confidence in their own abilities.

The school facility is often overlooked when considering field trips concerning health and safety. Yet the school directly affects each student. Think of all the aspects of health and safety that can be observed in any school: heating, lighting, acoustics, sanitation, water filtration, safety hazards, safety programs, fire prevention, and nutrition, just to name a few.

What areas can be visited? Why not consider the classrooms, hallways, science laboratories, home economics laboratory, vocational shops, swimming pool, boiler room, gymnasiums, stairways, cafeteria, kitchen, locker rooms, playground, athletic fields, guidance office, health clinic?

Let us assume that the behavioral objectives make a field trip desirable. How can students be involved in the planning? Suggestions:

1. If a problem such as "the identification of hazards" involves many different areas, a small coordinating committee can be formed. Various planning dyads can be set up to decide (a) where to visit, (b) how many students can be accommodated, (c) who needs to be contacted for permission and for answering their questions, (d) what specific questions do the students want to get answered, (e) what use can be made of the information gathered, (f) a unique way of thanking everyone who assisted the group.
2. A classroom teacher may want to spread the implementation of these plans over a period of time with his class. The specialist, with multiple sections, may choose to have each class plan for and visit different areas while compiling the data.
3. If it isn't feasible or desirable for an entire class to visit some areas, the class can divide into interest groups for visitation purposes.
4. Older students can be tapped as guides for areas where classes are in session. Other teachers are very cooperative and willing to suggest

students who are familiar with their specific area. Is the knowledge-able student a member of the visiting class? Why not make use of his knowledge?

When the problem being studied doesn't involve different areas and the space doesn't permit an entire class to make the visitation at one time, a field trip is not the desirable method. Under these circumstances, consider an individual project, a group project, or a guest speaker.

Guest Speaker. This method makes use of a person other than the regular teacher. The selection of the resource person is of utmost importance if the enrichment potential is to be achieved. The individual will of necessity have some expertise or experience potentially valuable to students. He must have the ability to communicate with students. Thus he must gear his vocabulary to the level of his audience without becoming patronizing.

Guest Speaker

Advantages	*Disadvantages*
Teacher:	Teacher:
1. Has access to materials not normally available.	1. May have problem scheduling speaker for all sections.
2. May obtain new ideas or new information.	2. Must prepare a "stand-by" plan to be used if speaker fails to appear.
3. Own expertise may be reinforced by guest.	
Student:	Student:
1. May observe a novel demonstration.	1. Is rarely involved except in a question and answer session after the presentation.
2. Has opportunity to receive another viewpoint.	2. May lose interest if speaker is boring or too technical.
3. May have interest stimulated.	
4. Experiences a change of "face" and of pace.	
5. May have own problems clarified.	
General:	General:
1. Students tend to accept information from a resource person that would be rejected if obtained from regular teacher.	1. Only one person's experience or point of view is given.

One of the common complaints of students is that insufficient time was permitted for asking questions about material they were interested in. How can the limitation of time be alleviated, and how can the experience be personalized for students? Modifications:

1. The class, groups, or dyads can develop the questions they wish to have answered.
2. Names of resource people who are capable of meeting the expressed needs, interests, or problems of the class can be developed.
3. The invitation to the selected speaker can specify that the class is interested in an informal question-and-answer session rather than a lecture.
4. Students can become involved in the follow-up contacts—in being hosts during the visit, and expressing their appreciation to the speaker.

The more that students are involved in the organization, the more they tend to look upon the guest as the speaker rather than merely a person brought in to entertain them. They know who he is, why he is there, and what they want from his visit. Some of our most outstanding speakers have been parents or personal acquaintances of the students. How often we fail to recognize the resources within our classes.

Laboratory Method (Skill Method). A program by which each student has an opportunity to develop some skill through practice.

Laboratory Method

Advantages	Disadvantages
Teacher:	Teacher:
1. Has opportunity to give individual assistance.	1. Must have facilities, equipment, and supplies.
2. Can immediately correct any misconceptions or errors.	2. More individual instruction is necessary.
3. Can easily assess competencies.	3. Must have sufficient skill himself.
Student:	Student:
1. Has opportunity to learn by doing.	1. Must have knowledge to participate.
2. Can work at own speed.	2. Lacking skill, may avoid participating.
3. Has time to perfect skill.	3. If unchallenged, may be a disciplinary problem.
4. Can receive personal assistance.	
5. Knows immediately when he is successful.	

Advantages	*Disadvantages*
General:	General:
1. Total participation is possible.	1. Process is time-consuming.
	2. Rarely possible with a large class.

Most teachers think of the laboratory method as applicable only to first-aid skills. They usually rationalize that they don't have enough space or equipment or supplies for their class.

There is no rule requiring all students to be doing the same thing at the same time. The creative facilitator improvises. He sets up a variety of stations (see Continuous Learning, p. 62) where students can work with the equipment available. Thus students can learn to operate the computer terminals, an overhead projector, a dry-mount press, a tape recorder, a slide projector, a film-strip projector, an opaque projector, a microscope, or whatever other equipment is available. In doing so, they may be observing a process or a skill to be practiced, preparing an audio or visual aid to present in class, or be involved in an experiment. The process may also have interdisciplinary transfer value.

Lecture Method. This is the most universally used teaching method, but also the least effective. It consists of a verbal presentation of a body of subject matter. It is an excellent example of one-way communication. The teacher is the only one who is active. The only indication a teacher receives of student understanding is nonverbal.

Lecture Method

Advantages	*Disadvantages*
Teacher:	Teacher:
1. Needs very few materials.	1. Can't be sure that students understand.
2. Can prepare lecture materials prior to school year without reference to any specific students.	2. Can be easily "turned off" by students.
3. Can use same material for multiple sections, which is time-saving.	3. Needs to be an excellent speaker to hold student attention.
4. Can easily "handle" large classes.	4. Often encourages disciplinary problems.
5. Can present large amount of content in short period of time.	5. Often lacks incentive to prepare current lecture material.

6. Has control over content discussed.
7. If non-creative finds this to be the easiest method to present content.

Student:
1. Doesn't have to prepare.
2. Can get class notes from others, if absent.
3. Can "loaf."
4. Learns to take notes.
5. Doesn't have to participate.
6. Can depend on teacher to do all the work.
7. Need take no responsibility for his own learning.

Student:
1. Is often bored by ineffectual presentation causing a form of hypnosis or potential disciplinary problem.
2. Has no opportunity for interaction with teacher or other students.
3. May not understand the vocabulary used.
4. Has no opportunity to develop or use his creativity.
5. Has no opportunity to disagree with expressed viewpoint.
6. Needs skill to take good notes.
7. Is often exposed to obsolete material.
8. Has only one chance to put information given into context.

General:
1. Can be used effectively for summary and review.
2. Inexpensive.
3. Special facilities are not needed.
4. Effective method of presenting factual material.
5. Everyone receives same information at the same time.
6. Lecture can be video-taped or duplicated for learning-center use by absent students.
7. Sets the stage for small group or independent study sessions to follow.

General:
1. Disadvantageous for the slower student.
2. Puts premium on taking notes quickly.
3. Content geared to instructor rather than student needs or interests.

Even with the many limitations inherent in the lecture method, it has a legitimate place in the classroom. There are times when cognitive input is essential.

Assume that one has decided that a lecture is the most desirable method to accomplish a purpose. There are some adaptations that can be made to minimize the normal disadvantages. Rather than attempt to hold student interest and attention with a straight lecture, try these techniques:

1. Design a lecturette that can be combined with another method permitting some type of interaction to occur.
2. Intersperse the lecture with thought-provoking questions that force students to apply immediately the information being presented.
3. Avoid being wedded to a lectern. Move around without pacing.
4. Make use of visual materials to illustrate or clarify. Judicious use of cartoon transparencies can aid in maintaining interest.
5. Use tension breakers—comments, stories, personal experiences applicable to the topic.

Project Method. Although this method usually is pursued by a small group, there may be individual projects (see Contract Method, p. 78). Occasionally, if an attempt is being made to improve a health or safety condition in the school or the community, an entire class may be involved. Some class time is usually devoted to project work in the early stages. The greater part of the time devoted to the project will, of necessity, be out of class.

Project Method

Advantages	*Disadvantages*
Teacher:	Teacher:
1. Is freed to give personalized assistance.	1. Has little opportunity to aid groups working on their own time.
2. Need not prepare lesson for periods students are working during class time.	2. Must be knowledgeable about resources.
3. Will have a minimum of disciplinary problems.	3. Needs to have reference materials available.
Student:	Student:
1. Learns to work with others.	1. May feel that project is busy work.
2. Can share ideas.	2. May have ideas that conflict with others.
3. Must make decisions.	3. May have unproductive member in group.
4. Can be creative.	
5. Can use own initiative.	
6. Can work at own speed.	

7. Tends to receive enrichment of knowledge from outside sources.
8. May be stimulated to further activity.
9. Has opportunity to apply concepts in a practical situation.
10. Learns by doing.
11. Receives organizational experience.

General:
1. Provides an opportunity for student improvement.
2. Promotes cooperative action.

4. May need to expend an inordinate amount of time for value received.
5. Can't always answer own questions.
6. May lack the abilities needed to be successful.
7. Those with talent may be favored.

General:
1. Evaluation tends to be subjective.
2. Is very time-consuming.
3. Summarization of important outcomes often lacking.

Facilitators attempt to avoid pursuing projects which are of limited interest or value to students. Unless there are important reasons for doing so, specific projects need not be assigned. Neither should students be manipulated into accepting projects that are of value principally to the teacher.

Within the framework of the behavioral objective, how can projects be originated? Suggestions:

1. Several possible projects may be suggested, with the option of student suggestions being added.
2. All suggestions may be generated by student groups through brainstorming techniques.
3. Projects may be pursued only when students have initiated the ideas. For example, many student groups have become personally involved in local paper- and glass-recycling programs, clean-up-the environment programs, and the like.

Question-and-Answer Method (Recitation; Textbook Study). This is one of the oldest teaching methods. It can be used very effectively. Unfortunately it is often misused and overused. The inexperienced teacher often employs it to assess whether the text has been read. Thus we have a "fencing-in" process that limits the responses to "what the textbook says." Used this way, it tends to become little more than a regurgitation of factual information. Moreover, the teacher may have little or no incentive to expand his own understanding beyond its present level.

Question-and-Answer Method

Advantages	Disadvantages

Teacher:

1. Can control what subject matter is discussed.
2. Can involve students who are reticent—inclined to avoid participation.
3. Can use in any facility.
4. Can adapt to any topic.
5. Knows which students have factual information.
6. Can prepare logical series of questions.
7. Can guide students to analytical thinking.
8. Can differentiate between known and unknown areas of information.

Student:

1. Has opportunity to participate.
2. Can challenge teacher.
3. Can express personal opinion.
4. Can avoid participating by not volunteering.
5. Always has the source available when the material is textbook-based.

General:

1. Misunderstanding can be corrected immediately.
2. Wide participation can be fostered.
3. Is useful for reviewing factual content.

Teacher:

1. Tends to teach subject matter rather than students.
2. Tends to become discouraged with nonresponsive classes.
3. Must carefully preplan questions.
4. Is easily sidetracked.
5. May develop an argumentative session with more aggressive students.

Student:

1. Isn't encouraged to go beyond one source of information.
2. Is often bored.
3. Is often embarrassed if he fails to know "right" answer.
4. Will not risk subsequent embarrassment if he is "put down."
5. Will resent over-participation by "favored" students.
6. Isn't encouraged to be creative.

General:

1. Can't be used effectively with a large class.
2. Tends to be ineffective with slow learners.
3. Text used as source is often obsolete.

The use of the Question-and-Answer method need not be limited to the recall of facts. Facilitators will utilize questions in many different ways.

Suggestions:

1. Pose thought-provoking questions having multiple answers.
2. Pose questions having no known answers.
3. Develop questions in the affective domain that are open-ended. Since these are based on individual values, opinions, attitudes, there can be no one correct answer.
4. Devise questions that will encourage students to apply their knowledge in practical situations.
5. Encourage students to develop their questioning abilities. This technique encourages improved class discussions.
6. Avoid using Question-and-Answer as the only method for a class period. It can be an effective way of leading into other methods, including small group discussion, role play, or demonstration.
7. It can be just as effectively used following another method to evaluate or to focus upon the important facets brought out.

Role-Play Method (Sociodrama). With this method a group of students is given a situation and is assigned to the needed roles. Each student formulates his lines as he goes along, based on his own ideas of how his character would act in the situation and what the other characters say in their roles.

Role-Play Method

Advantages	*Disadvantages*
Teacher:	Teacher:
1. Receives immediate feedback from class.	1. Needs to structure situations that are applicable to student lives.
2. Learns more about student attitudes.	2. Needs skill to extract learnings.
3. Tends to have a more relaxed atmopshere for following discussion.	3. Has no way of knowing how the role-play will develop.
4. Can provide a contrived purposeful activity.	4. May have difficulty evaluating.
Student:	Student:
1. Has opportunity to be creative.	1. May, if timid, hesitate to become involved.
2. Tends to enjoy participating as well as seeing others' interpretations.	2. May be unaware of purpose and/or meaning.
3. Tends to become emotionally involved in situation.	3. Who is aggressive may get to participate constantly.
4. Has opportunity to hear opposing viewpoints.	4. May be bored if the situation is not well done.

Advantages	Disadvantages

5. Develops confidence in talking in front of a group.
6. Has opportunity to express emotions and feelings.
7. Can develop empathy for others.

General:
1. It is student-centered.
2. Role-playing holds the attention of students.

General:
1. It is time-consuming.
2. Relatively few can participate.

This method can be extremely effective in a variety of areas. It is usually considered for use only with concepts relating to family or social situations. Imaginative facilitators have found that role-playing can be of value when applied to growth and development, to utilization of health products, and even to disease and environment. In these instances, role-players are the body or body part, the health product, the disease, or the pollutant.

Small Group Discussion (Buzz Groups). This is an organizational technique used in a normal-sized class. Depending on the purpose, groups of from two to eight persons meet together in a designated section of the classroom. It may be desirable for the groups to be composed of both sexes or of the same sex. All groups may be discussing the same topic or each group may have a different topic. The discussions may range from brainstorming to problem-solving. Whatever the purpose, it is important that some method be designed that will permit all groups to share their ideas with the rest of the class.

Small Group Discussion

Advantages	Disadvantages

Teacher:
1. Has time to get involved with all groups.
2. Can give more attention to groups needing assistance.
3. Can involve more students in the discussion.
4. Spends less time in planning.
5. Has opportunity to develop rapport with students in a less formal atmosphere.

Teacher:
1. Needs skill to coordinate diverse opinions.
2. Has no control over what is said.
3. Needs to develop skill in supervising.

Student:
1. Gets to know other students in the class.
2. Learns to work with others.
3. Can share own knowledge and ideas with others.
4. Will feel more responsibility for contributing to the discussion.
5. Learns to express himself.
6. Has opportunity to develop leadership skills.
7. Can gain confidence through acceptance of his ideas.
8. Learns from others.
9. Tends to retain more.
10. Feels secure in smaller groups.
11. Learns to evaluate materials and ideas.
12. Develops organizational ability.

General:
1. Provides workable method of breaking down a large class.
2. Gets everyone involved.
3. Provides a change of pace.
4. Total class benefits from other group findings.

Student:
1. May be overpowered by aggressive group members.
2. May have difficulty working with others.

General:
1. Is more time-consuming.
2. May be a "pooling of ignorance."
3. Is difficult to evaluate.
4. Digression is easy.
5. The noise level is higher.
6. Teacher may "over-use" this technique.

Team Teaching. The team teaching concept is usually referred to as a "teaching method." This is a misnomer, as team teaching is an administrative and organizational plan. The team will choose and execute the teaching methods to be employed in the classroom.

In all probability the preprofessional health educator will participate in a team teaching experience, if not initially in his career, soon thereafter. Team teaching is no longer categorized as something new and bright on the horizon. This concept has been in existence for many years. But each year more and more educators are recognizing the exciting potential value of team teaching in helping to expedite the ultimate objective of all education —student learning.

The term "team teaching" can be interpreted in many ways by persons who have participated in it. Basically it is a cooperative planning, facilitating, and evaluating effort utilizing the talents of two or more facilitators to reach the objectives of a teaching/learning concept. The same fundamentals that go into making any kind of a team successful are essential in team teaching. A member of a teaching team should demonstrate:

1. Cooperation
    a. A willingness to work together.
    b. A recognition of the talents and weaknesses of the team members.
    c. A willingness to delegate responsibility to team members relative to their strongest competencies.
    d. Diplomacy—recognition of personality differences among team members.
    e. A willingness to work, to accept, and to execute responsibility and leadership.

2. Flexibility
    a. A willingness to accept innovations—to continue learning.
    b. A willingness to accept and give help—to accept and give constructive criticism and suggestions to team members.
    c. A willingness to accept change and make adjustments to change in his facilitating role.
    d. Ability to recognize a job well done by a team member and to compliment him on it.

3. Planning
    a. Planning—leadership in his area of responsibility, but an open-mindedness toward the ideas and creative talents of his co-workers.
    b. A willingness to plan objectives and learning experiences bearing in mind that all plans must be flexible to meet the needs of individual classes or students.

Since team teaching necessitates organizational planning by administrators (many books have been written about the various plans used throughout the country), these processes will not be discussed in this book. It should be pointed out, however, that most plans include some common threads of continuity, such as:

1. Some form of flexible scheduling;
2. A form of pupil-grouping;
3. A built-in time for cooperative planning by team members; and
4. The utilization of time, space, personnel, and media appropriate to the task involved.

The preprofessional should also be made aware of some of the advantages and disadvantages of this team teaching process before he assumes his position of "facilitator of learning."

Team Teaching

Advantages

Teacher:

1. May expand creativity horizons.
2. May be motivated to update his knowledge in subject area.
3. May learn new techniques and methodology from co-workers.
4. May strengthen his own communication skills.
5. Can become more student-oriented in group planning.
6. May become more effective in conceptual planning, the writing of behavioral objectives, and evaluative techniques.
7. Will probably get to know more students well through small group interactions and as a result be able to assess individual needs.
8. Will have more flexibility in combining classes or interchanging students with other team members for specific purposes.
9. Will have scheduled time for team planning and assessment.
10. Is not dependent upon his own subjective judgment in evaluation of student performance.

Disadvantages

Teacher:

1. May feel threatened in being forced to work with a team rather than autonomously.
2. May be reluctant to change from traditional methods of teaching.
3. May feel resistant to giving time necessary for efficient planning and additional responsibility.
4. May be forced to plan and execute large group presentations (which may be an unfamiliar experience).
5. May feel insecure in having team members observe his teaching.
6. May feel embarrassed if a presentation "bombs."
7. May feel uncomfortable changing his role from that of teacher-leader to facilitator.
8. May find some members of team are not committed to the team teaching concept.
9. May lack flexibility needed to accommodate differing viewpoints.
10. May feel resentful at the division of leadership within the team.
11. May be sensitive to constructive criticism.

Advantages	*Disadvantages*

11. May discover that the blending of talents and interests will enlarge competencies and minimize weaknesses.
12. Will grow professionally through team interaction and experience.
13. May involve more community resources in student learning-experiences through more contacts within the team.
14. Will find opportunities for developing a team library of resource and audio-visual materials.
15. Will be able to assess, with team members, the strengths and weaknesses of the program and make appropriate revisions.

12. May get "hung up" to philosophical differences regarding issues, procedures, and/or evaluations.
13. Work load may be increased.

Student:

1. Will have the benefit of exposure to more than one teacher.
2. Will develop a closer relationship with team teachers through interaction activities.
3. May have more opportunity and motivation, through team planning, to "learn to learn."
4. Will feel a change from being "talked to" to being guided in learning.
5. Will be exposed to more varied and relevant learning experiences.
6. Will derive the benefit of having a variety of evaluative activities measuring his performance.
7. Will have his learning performance evaluated by more

Student:

1. Must communicate and relate to more than one teacher.
2. Must, of necessity, develop more independent learning skills.
3. Cannot rely solely upon objective or subjective "regurgitation-type" evaluation.
4. May feel an added pressure in assuming more responsibility for learning.
5. May feel incompetent or uneasy in small group interaction activities.
6. May rely on his peers who are verbally more competent.
7. Will have less opportunity to be sedentary in learning.
8. If involved in his learning, must help build up his competencies.

than one teacher; the influence of possible personality conflicts will thus be lessened.

8. May himself be involved in his own evaluation and that of his peers.

9. Due to involvement in learning may be less tempted to be disruptive.

10. Through sharing an understanding of the behavioral objectives, will know what he is expected to learn.

11. May become more adept in discussion and decision-making.

12. Through interaction with peers and teaching team, may make value judgments that will stand him in good stead throughout his life.

13. May be grouped and evaluated according to his ability.

14. Will have less opportunity for failure if he actively participates in his learning.

General:

1. Upgrades the quality of teaching/learning, of utmost importance in the age of accountability.

2. Opens other avenues of curriculum and general school innovations.

3. Promotes more effective staff utilization.

4. The use of nonteaching personnel may supplement a teaching team.

9. May feel uncomfortable in the interchange of groups among team teachers.

General:

1. Members new to a team teaching situation may need training in the new role.

2. Unequal participation by team members (leading role vs. supporting role) may prove a difficult adjustment to some members.

3. Team members need to develop skills in new teaching techniques.

4. Teams must recognize the

5. Will make possible a more effective use of libraries, learning centers, and other facilities.
6. Will probably stimulate and strengthen professional growth on the part of individual team members.
7. Cooperation and flexibility among team members may carry over into more total staff harmony.
8. "Team" aspect of teaching may strengthen a weak teacher.
9. New teachers with fresh ideas and enthusiasm may serve as a catalyst to the team.
10. Experienced teachers may add guidance and stability to a team.
11. Gives teachers the opportunity to try new things. "Nothing ventured, nothing gained" attitude takes hold.
12. May give the total staff a sense of direction and pride in a job well done.
13. May meet the learning needs of students more effectively.

need to update and revise content, objectives, and techniques constantly.
5. Team teaching demands great effort on the part of everyone involved.
6. Team teaching necessitates the skillful development of flexible guidelines.
7. Successful team teaching demands involvement by both teachers and students.
8. Final decisions and judgments regarding content, learning activities, and evaluation rest with the team and not with an individual member—no focal point of responsibility.

Team Planning

One of the most important phases of team teaching is the planning sessions. In most instances the team members have a common meeting time built into their teaching schedule when they can rap together on all the ramifications of their endeavors. Since team teaching is a complex process, the planning session needs to be organized in order to be effective. Organization implies leadership. Two possible types of leadership may emerge on a team. One is hierarchical, wherein one teacher assumes an administrative role. This teacher may be appointed by a school administrator or a department head, or he may be chosen by a consensus of the team members. The other possibility is a system of cooperative leader-

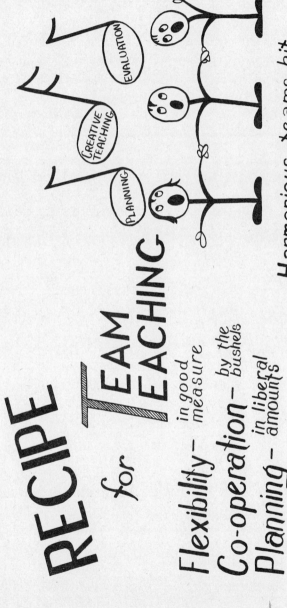

RECIPE for TEAM TEACHING

Flexibility— in good measure
Co-operation— by the bushels
Planning— in liberal amounts

Blend carefully, and serve proudly to students who hunger for learning at its best.

Harmonious teams hit all three notes.

Lois Lehman
— Drawing by Laurel Wilcox

ship where no leader is designated, decisions being reached through the interactions of team members. Both types of leadership have advantages and disadvantages.

Team Teaching Leadership Styles

Advantages	Disadvantages
Hierarchical:	Hierarchical:
1. Decision-making is more readily expedited.	1. Team members may feel inhibited in their creativity.
2. Responsibilities of team members can be more clearly defined and delegated.	2. The individual team members may have philosophical conflicts with the leader.
3. The team leader can exhibit guidance and direction to the team.	
Cooperative Leadership:	Cooperative Leadership:
1. Leadership is assumed by the initiating teacher.	1. Decision-making may be tedious and nebulous.
2. There is a potential for individual growth through intensive interaction.	2. Assessments by the team of an individual's strengths and weaknesses may cause friction.
3. All members contribute to the program at all times.	3. This system may be more demanding of each team member.

In a team meeting there are two clearly defined roles for individual members. One is that of the "initiating" teacher who is responsible for planning all phases of his assigned area of curriculum. He formulates the behavioral objectives, designs the learning and evaluative activities, plans for the resources to be utilized, and sees that the concept is being developed.

The "supporting" teachers, although not responsible for the planning, carry through the scheme of the initiator in the actual facilitating. They evaluate the results of the plan together (and possibly with the students), and share their experiences after a particular concept has been completed.

It is at the team meeting where students' needs, the strengths and weaknesses in a plan or in its execution, pupil performance, and future plans are discussed. There it is decided which team member will be the "initiating" teacher for a particular concept with a particular grade level. Thus every team member will fill this role from time to time, supported by others on the team.

Conclusion

In team teaching a variety of teaching methods are used in the development of concepts. The facilitator is not locked into using a limited number of techniques. Each has the chance to explore, to attempt, to change. Very little opportunity exists to become self-satisfied because planning and evaluating are ongoing and dynamic. Team members soon discover that revising, adjusting, rearranging, or even abandoning plans is a continuous process. This is "facilitator growth."

7

MEDIA UNLIMITED

In this era of advanced technology, the variety of available teaching-learning aids is unlimited. For teachers who have been in the field for twenty years or more, the profusion of aids can be overwhelming. For today's preprofessional, who has grown up with these developments, it is hard to visualize *not* having these resources available.

The preprofessional normally has a distinct advantage in having one or more excellent undergraduate audio visual courses available to him. Here he can develop his own competencies in using the available equipment and in devising materials to enhance his future teaching. Certification standards in many states require an audio visual course for all education majors. For students in states not requiring it, such a course is recommended. It will prove to be highly beneficial.

Although not every school has all of the books, media, and equipment a facilitator might desire, federal funding programs have made it possible for most schools to provide the basic media needed. The Title III program of the National Defense Education Act (NDEA, 1957) provided funds for Instructional Media. The Title II program of the Elementary and Secondary Education Act (1965) made funds available for library books.

Facilitators who make effective use of the books, media, and equipment on hand, and can prove the desirability of additional media and equipment, will have little difficulty in adding needed media and equipment as funds become available. The more facilitators who request an item, the higher the priority that item will have in a budget.

Current methods textbooks continue to emphasize the importance of using multi media materials and equipment to improve *teaching* effectiveness. One cannot dispute that the judicious blending of methods and media will enhance teaching skills. The implication is, however, that the teacher secure and utilize the selected media. This relegates the student to the role of inactive receiver and, as a result, minimizes the probability that facilitators will consider involving students in this aspect of their learning. Again the plea is made—focus on students! Keep in mind Edgar Dale's comment, "We do not use any one medium of communication in isolation. Rather we use many instructional materials to help the student conceptualize his experience so that he can deal with it effectively."[1]

Textbooks. Teachers usually consider a textbook an absolutely necessary basic tool. When one views the reality of typical school situations, however, a book as *the* text becomes less than desirable. The purchasing of a book or an elementary series entails a large expenditure for a school system. After this expenditure there is no opportunity to change to more appropriate books as they become available. Thus it is not uncommon to find books with copyright dates of from eleven to twenty years ago still in use. For a field as dynamic as health education this is a tragedy. Let us assume that one has selected a "best" new textbook. By the time it is written, edited, printed, and reaches the public, it tends to be partially dated. Rarely does a month pass without bringing scientific discoveries, additional information, and medical breakthroughs. In addition, changing attitudes within communities often make it acceptable to discuss problems in the classroom that previously were taboo. As a result, many relatively new textbooks either contain no information in these areas or treat them very superficially.

To eliminate the problems inherent in a basic textbook, facilitators should consider using multitexts as references. As new books are published, it is comparatively easy to secure ten copies. To this end, there are several possible approaches that may be used. Library funds may be made available. Federal funding, such as the previously mentioned Elementary and Secondary Education Act, Title II, may exist for the purchase of library books. If school funds are not divided by departments, administrators tend to approve such small expenditures. If there is a departmental budget, one can designate an item for reference books. Thus, over a period of time, an excellent health education library section can be developed. When such a section is housed in the school library, the books are available to all students. When various books are needed in the classroom or in the Learning Center, they can be placed on a cart and wheeled in.

In addition to the obvious value of having current texts, there are other advantages in this approach: (1) Students have several sources of information. This assists them in reading critically and decreases the tendency to accept statements as fact "because the text says so." (2) Books geared to different reading levels can be secured. Students with reading difficulties as

1. Edgar Dale, *Audiovisual Methods in Teaching,* 3rd ed. (New York: The Dryden Press, Inc., 1969), p. 133.

well as honors students have references available to meet their capabilities. (3) Multiple sources give a variety of viewpoints rather than the single viewpoint of a common textbook.

Adhesion Boards. The great variety of surfaces to which instructional material can be attached fall into this category. Included are the standard bulletin board, the peg board, the magnetic board, and such cloth-backed boards as have a napped surface (commonly referred to as felt or flannel boards, although they utilize burlap, velvet, suede, or duveteen equally well). The Hook n' Loop®[2] board is the only cloth-backed board that can be attached permanently to a wall area perpendicularly. The backing cloth consists entirely of tiny loops, while the special tapes that must be glued to the back of the mounts consist of tiny hooks. Thus the surface has the strength and tenacity to support three-dimensional objects up to fifty pounds in weight.

Bulletin boards, magnetic boards, and Hook n' Loop® boards tend to be permanently installed. Although peg boards, flannel boards, and felt boards are usually portable, the other surfaces are equally effective in portable form. Almost anything that can be displayed on one surface can be mounted on any other. The exception is real objects, the weight or bulk of which make the Hook n' Loop® board, the magnetic board, or the peg board the most logical display surfaces. Objects will adhere to these surfaces without danger of falling off.

Portable boards are most effective when utilized for individual or small group study.

As one visits classrooms, it is strikingly evident how rarely adhesion boards are effectively used. They are often receptacles for unattractive, dated displays of materials unrelated to classroom activities. Our observation has been that elementary teachers consistently make the most effective use of the available display space.

It is extremely easy to rationalize ineffective use. One can say, ". . . but I don't have any artistic ability," or "When do I have time to do this in addition to everything else?" In answer to the first, one doesn't need artistic ability. In answer to the second, the creation of bulletin-board displays can be meaningful learning activities for individual students or groups of students.

There are some simple guidelines that will, if followed, result in very eye-appealing exhibits:

1. Choose a topic.
2. Look for ideas. Good sources are radio and television commercials, the comics in newspapers, cartoons, magazine advertisements, etc.

---

2. Originally registered by Charles Mayer Studios, Inc. Akron, Ohio. Now available through school supply houses, art and commercial art dealers.

3. Develop a short title that has an instant message for observers.
4. Plan the layout. Here again, one of the best sources for effective layouts is magazine ads. Blank sheets the size of the material to be displayed can be manipulated on a table or floor to visualize the effect on the board space. Use string to outline the exact dimensions of the board to be used.
5. Choose the color scheme to be used. A general rule of thumb is to use no more than three colors.
6. Since most board surfaces are neutral in color and often soiled, a background material should be used to provide contrast for the material to be displayed. Consider burlap, construction paper, white wrapping paper from a roll, or crepe paper. For specific displays, maps, sheet music, and newspaper pages have been very effective.
7. If metal-backed chalkboards are being used for magnetic bulletin boards or if a Hook n' Loop® board is available, no other background material should be used.
8. Prepare the display material. Photos or pictures can be dry-mounted on construction paper for contrast.
9. If it is desirable to preserve display material for future use, consider lamination. This is more expensive, but items can be cleaned and do not tear or fade.
10. Use an opaque projector to enlarge any drawing, character, figure, etc. Place the figure to be reproduced on the projector platform. Using masking tape, attach the material to be used on the wall. Project the image on the material. Adjust the distance until the desired size is reached. Trace the projected image in pencil on the wall-mounted backing. Add color at a table to prevent smear or bleed-through to the wall surface. Felt tip markers, which are available in a wide range of colors and varied thicknesses, come in very handy at this point.
11. For the caption, use letters large enough to be read from a distance. Stencils of various sizes and styles are available. Both 1½" and 3" sizes are practical. Commercial letters for magnetic boards and Hook n' Loop® boards are more practical and cheaper over a period of time.
12. Use a border that contrasts with the background material to frame the display. It adds a definitive finishing touch.

By following these guidelines, it becomes a simple task to assist individuals or groups of students to construct bulletin board displays that stimulate interest, encourage learning, and develop creativity.

The displays need not be limited to the classroom. The hallways, cafeteria, and study halls have exhibition cases and bulletin boards that can be utilized for displays of interest to the total school population.

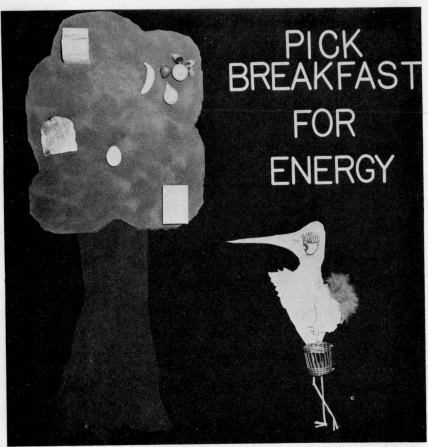

— Sue Ledyard, Kent State University

Note the photos of student-constructed bulletin boards. The creativity shown by students in implementing their ideas is quite evident.

If a bulletin board is going to be used only to brighten up the decor, we suggest that it be a teacher project. If, however, it is to be a learning activity, we recommend that it be a student project. Not only will a student learn how to create a good display but he gains in other ways: (1) He has a feeling of achievement; (2) He can evaluate his own product; (3) He receives evaluations from his peers with suggestions for improvement; (4) His product is utilized in the learning process; (5) He has provided a learning tool for others; (6) The praise he receives from others makes him feel successful; (7) He has the opportunity to develop a psychomotor skill.

A suggested tool for evaluating bulletin boards is given on p. 138.

Transparencies. Tranparencies are acetate visuals to be used with overhead projectors. They may be purchased completely prepared from school suppliers or made entirely by hand. Thermographic or Diazo processing from commercial or hand-made masters can also be done.

Commercially made transparencies are technically of excellent quality, are in color, and are the most expensive. Some commercial transparencies are made with imbedded polarized strips. By using a light-polarizing attachment on the projector, movement, such as circulation of blood, can be produced. The movement is controlled by the speed of the spinning attachment.

Transparency masters are less expensive and are also of good quality. Another advantage they have is that as many identical copies as desired can be made from the master just for the cost of the material. Various

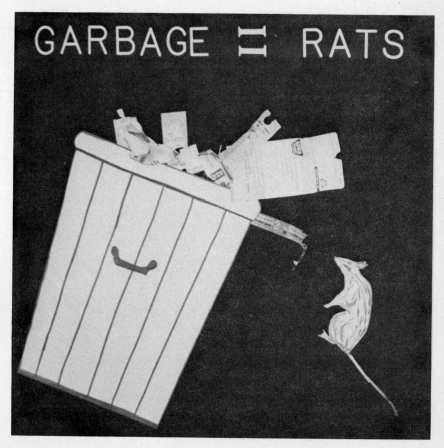

— Janet Falbo, Kent State University

commercial companies produce packets of loose-leaf binders of masters. Tear-out masters are published in some professional journals and in a few soft-bound professional books. They may be designed to be duplicated by the Diazo process or the thermographic process. The Diazo process uses colored acetate which when processed produces color. Although thermographic transparencies are black on a clear acetate, color may be added after processing. To do this, trace the design desired on a sensitive color sheet, remove the backing material, and press in place on the transparency.

The hand-made transparency is the least expensive and the most time-consuming to produce. Unless one has drawing ability, it will also be of the poorest quality.

Unfortunately, all the visual material a facilitator may desire to have in transparency form does not exist from a commercial source. Thus he either must have a production service available in the school system or he must make it himself.

Quite commonly one finds material in another form that would be useful as a transparency. If production services are available, it is simply a matter of deciding what content one wants on the base and on each overlay. The production specialist processes the requisition and charges the department budget for the materials used.

When the facilitator must produce his own, it is suggested that he avoid acetate ink unless he is skilled in its use. Felt tip markers prepared for use on acetate are available either in permanent nonsoluble form or water-soluble form. The use of water-soluble markings permits the acetate to be reused.

There are easier methods that can be used:

For a drawing or diagram:

1. Trace with a No. 2 pencil on smooth bond paper.
2. Process this master with acetate through the thermographic desk copier.
3. Use dry transfer letters for labeling.
4. Use adhesive-backed color cellophane for color, if desired.

For a chart:

1. Type copy on bond using a high-carbon ribbon and large type. (Special education and primary departments have this style of typewriter.)
2. If high-carbon ribbon is not available, some other methods can be used.
   a. Deliberately place a sheet of carbon paper in reverse against the back of the bond paper upon which you will type your material.

This will print a reverse image on the back of the original and thus supply the carbon image needed for the thermographic desk copier.

1. Either keep the bond paper and carbon paper together as a unit as they come out of the typewriter and process it in the thermographic copier, or
2. Carefully remove the carbon paper and replace it with a clean sheet. Process it in the desk copier. Either method will reduce smearing the carbon image and will avoid getting the copier roller dirty.
   b. An easier method, but one resulting in a lower-quality transparency, is to make a Xerox copy of the typed copy. Then process this master with the acetate through the thermographic desk copier.

Incidently, these masters can also be processed by a desk copier to produce a master to be used on a liquid duplicator. Thus, without retyping, one can provide handout charts, diagrams, or sketches for the class.

A ready supply of blank acetates and grease pencils can come in very handy for temporary use. These can be used and reused by students as well as by facilitators. Students can prepare visual presentations to report the progress or the decisions made by their particular groups to the class. The transparencies are also effective focal points for clarification or emphasis.

Transparencies have an advantage over the same material placed on the chalkboard. If the material needs to be used for more than one class period or in another room, it is readily available and need not be recopied. When one is finished, it is easily cleaned by rubbing with a facial tissue or soft cloth. Thus a small number of acetates can be constantly recycled.

Over a period of time a facilitator accumulates a permanent file of transparencies. The ones appropriate to a concept can be used by the facilitator or by students. Placed in the Learning Center, they are available to students engaged in Independent Study, a group project, or a Continuous-Learning Program.

Dry Mounts and Laminations. Preserving short articles, pictures, or photos for display purposes is most easily done by either dry mounting or laminating.

Dry mounting is accomplished by using dry-mount tissue, which is extruded shellac and looks like waxed paper. It is a simple process of using heat to bond a picture to a background material neatly and firmly. The bumps or spots frequent with paste or glue do not occur.

1. Cut the tissue to the size of the object to be mounted.
2. Tack it, so that it doesn't slip, with a tacking iron or an electric iron.

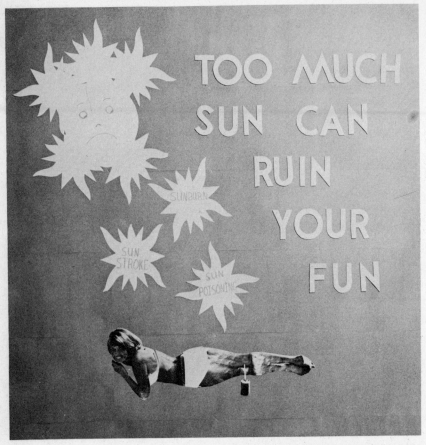

— Carol Campbell, Kent State University

3. Place the object on a piece of construction paper and again tack it in place.
4. Place the mounted picture between a doubled sheet of clear, unprinted paper. This keeps any tissue from sticking to the press.
5. Place the covered object on the platform of a dry-mount press. Close the lid and heat.
6. An electric iron is a good substitute if no dry-mount press is available.

Laminating is the use of mylar film to permanently protect a mounted or unmounted page, article, or picture. It can be wiped clean, will not tear, fray, or sun-fade. Grease pencils or water-soluble felt-tipped pens can also be used over the laminated material to add information that can be removed later.

1. If the sheet has not been mounted, place it in the press for a few seconds to remove any moisture.
2. Cut enough mylar film to cover both sides. If only one side is covered, the sheet will curl.
3. Place between a double-folded sheet of clear, unprinted paper.
4. Put the covered object on the platform of the dry-mount press. Close the lid and heat.
5. Remove. If not completely bonded, return to the press.
6. Any air bubbles can be pricked with a pin and reheated.
7. Remove from the cover and trim any excess film from the edges.

Laminated pictures are easily filed and can be handled without permanent damage. Any soil is easily wiped off. Mylar film is more expensive than dry-mount tissue. The determination whether to and how to protect an object depends upon the use to which it will be put. Valuable or frequently used materials can be both mounted and laminated to prolong their period of usefulness.

Tear-Sheet Files. Excellent articles pertinent to health education appear frequently in current magazines. An article can be a valuable resource for the class. The facilitator may choose to place such articles in a booklet form for reference purposes.

Usually the article is of temporary value. If so, it is recommended that it be processed by the most inexpensive method. The only cost involved is for the poster board and binding tape.

1. Remove the staples from the center fold of the magazine and remove the double pages containing the article. Do *not* tear out.
2. Cut opposite page ½" from the center fold. This will permit pages to open without any loss of text or picture when bound.
3. For the front and back covers, cut poster board slightly larger than the article plus the half-inch.
4. Staple the article in three or four places to the back cover.
5. Put the title on the front cover. If it is printed on the magazine cover, dry mount the cover or the pertinent portion of it on the poster board.
6. Staple the front cover to the article and the back cover.
7. Fold the front cover back, even with the center fold of the article.
8. Bind with adhesive-backed colored tape.

When the article is of more permanent usefulness, one should consider a process that is more expensive:

1. Prepare the article the same as directed in #1, 2, 3 above.
2. Cut strips of dry-mount tissue slightly narrower than the ½" selvage.
3. Cut poster board for covers.
4. Put the title on the front cover.

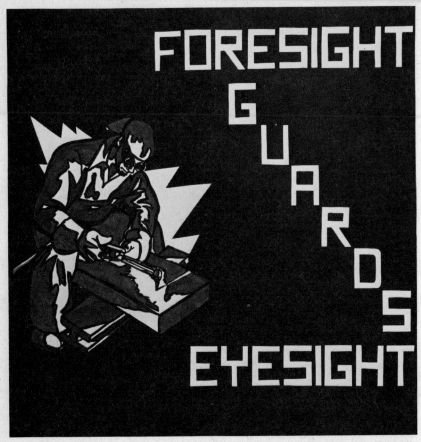

— Thomas Burick, Kent State University

5. Dry-mount the first page and/or back pages of the article on the in-
    side surfaces of the covers, dependent on whether the article begins
    and ends on a right-hand page.
6. Laminate each page and both covers, using a dry-mount press.
7. Tack each strip of dry-mount tissue to the selvage. Seal with a dry-
    mount press one page at a time until the booklet is complete.
8. Fold the front cover even with the selvage.
9. Bind with adhesive-backed colored tape.

   Although laminating each page is more expensive, it permanently
protects the article.

   Accumulating a series of tear-sheet files adds up-to-date reference
materials for student use. The articles are easily filed, no space being taken
up by the unneeded remainder of the magazine. In addition, those files not
of permanent value can be discarded as they become dated.

Tapes: Reels and Cassettes. Commercial tapes relevant to health education concepts are available. Recently cassettes have become more popular, probably because of the lower cost of a recorder, and the considerable ease of using. Since no threading is necessary, the likelihood of breaking a tape is greatly reduced.

In addition to commercial tapes, facilitators can make use of "home made" tapes. The possibilities are unlimited. Consider the practicality of the following suggestions:

1. "Getting to know you." Use a different cassette for each class. Set the recorder up in a corner of the room with the microphone ready to be switched on. Pose one question, such as "What one thing would you like to have me know about you?" or "If I were to ask your best friend what you were *really* like, what one thing would you hope your friend would tell me?" While the class continues, students go to the station setup. They record their names and their answers to the question.
2. When students interview an outside expert, record the interview for reporting to the class.
3. When students make a survey, record the responses.
4. Record a guest speaker. The tape can be used for those classes which were unable to hear that guest speak. It can also be placed in the Learning Center for students who were absent.
5. Record a radio or TV program of interest to a class.
6. Record health advertisements for discussion and evaluation of their claims.
7. Representatives from a class plan and record a message of appreciation to a guest speaker or to the host of a field trip.
8. Large group lectures by the facilitator may be taped and placed in the Learning Center or library for use by students who were absent on the presentation day. Since most small group learning activities usually follow the large group and are directly related, there is no excuse for students to be unprepared.

Models. Commercial models of all the parts of the body are available. They are expensive, but very useful for individual or small group work, as most of them can be disassembled for closer study. Duplication can sometimes be avoided by coordination with the Science Department. Less expensive plastic models in kit form are also available. Putting them together can be a valuable learning experience.

Frequently one has students who are interested in constructing models and have the skill to do so—e.g., a tooth model of balsa wood, sawed in half and the component parts painted. Another example is the G-Sled illustrated on p. 116. Plans for its construction are on p. 117.

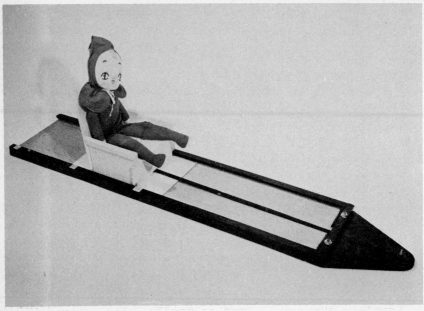

G-Sled
— Photo by Lawrence Rubens
— Rodney Lopick, Kent State University

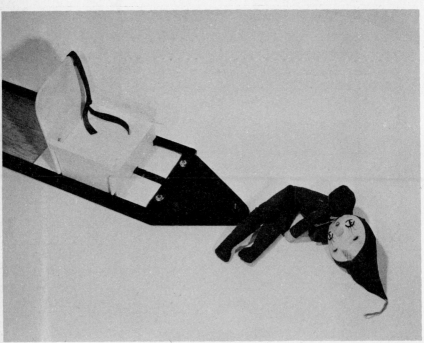

G-Sled
— Photo by Lawrence Rubens
— Rodney Lopick, Kent State University

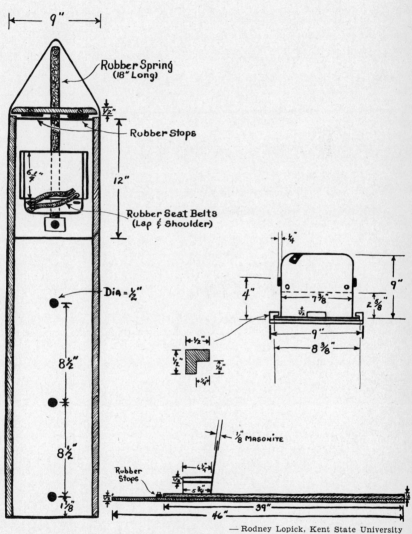

— Rodney Lopick, Kent State University
—Drawing by Laurel Wilcox

Construction Plans for G-Sled

Other media to consider are plaster, papier-mâché, plastic clay, Styrofoam, and Plexiglas. The Art and Industrial Arts departments are invaluable to both students and facilitators for ideas and assistance. Consider the values of inter- or multi-disciplinary activities.

Realia. The actual objects lend realism to classroom activities. Facilitators can frequently secure defective products from the manufacturer at no cost. Students tend to be very much interested in seeing and handling such items as heart valves, artificial eyes, intrauterine devices, hearing aids, contact lenses, a dental bridge, a crown, or a brace. A nearby slaughter house will gladly provide animal parts, such as hinge or ball and socket joints, heart, tongue, or eye, from a cow, a pig, or a sheep. Because of the size of real objects, usage is most effective with individuals or in small groups.

Shade Charts. Commercial anatomical charts are available, but also very expensive. Where funds are limited and this type of aid is needed, window shades can be substituted very inexpensively. An advantage of the home-made chart is that only the amount of labeling of value to the students need be put on the chart.

All that is necessary is:

1. To find a diagram that suits the purpose;
2. Project it on the shade using an opaque projector;
3. Outline the diagram;
4. Color and add the labels desired.
5. Cut and stain a scrap piece of wood ½″ thick, 4″ wide, slightly longer than the shade, to serve as hanger.
6. Attach the shade brackets to the hanger.
7. Screw two cup hooks in the top edge for hanging.

When buying the shade, ask for some samples of the shade material. Test the brand of felt tip pen on the scrap material. Not all types will work on all shade surfaces. Large, dry transfer letters make a very professional-looking job, save time if one is not adept at free-hand lettering, and can be seen from a distance.

One clever student constructed a long, slender box large enough to hold several shades and display material. It was approximately 36″ long, 5″ wide, and 6″ tall. The shade brackets were installed inside each end. When the top was lifted, a long dowel was inserted through two brackets— one attached on the upper middle of the lid, the other on the lower middle of the box back. The dowel had a small nail about one inch from the top. The dowel served as a support when the shade was pulled up. The nail held it in place. One shade was an anatomical chart. A second had Hook n' Loop® material attached, which gave the student an adhesion "board." He had prepared a genetic display which included male and

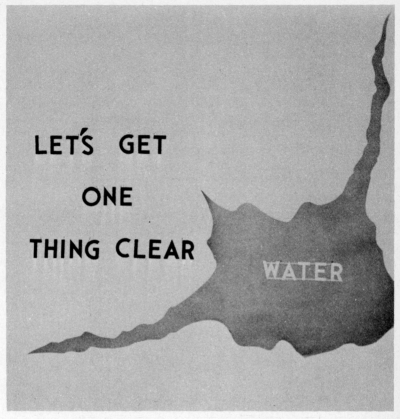

LET'S GET

ONE

THING CLEAR

WATER

— Earl Menges, Kent State University

female paper dolls and materials to clarify dominant and recessive characteristics. The box was large enough to store additional shades as they were prepared. The handle on the outside top surface provided ease of portability, a feature that makes it very practical, particularly when classes meet in a variety of classrooms.

Suitcase Exhibits. This is a term loosely applied to any display enclosed either in an actual suitcase or in a self-made carrying case. It is portable and can contain a permanent display or surfaces where displays can be changed. Suggestions:

1. An inexpensive suitcase lined with Styrofoam was made into a very attractive drug facsimile exhibit. The lining had pockets cut out to hold the items. It was then colored to provide contrast for display items. Empty gelatin capsules were painted with felt tip pens, and various proprietary pills were added in the proper size and shape. A thick sheet of plastic covered the display and was studded with straight pins around the edges.

2. "Suitcases" of scrap wood or the poorest grade of ⅜" plywood have been very effective. Painting the plywood a dark color keeps the knots from being distracting and provides a background for a permanent display. Any type of display that can be reproduced in wood can be mounted and colored. Lengths of colored, coated wire can be used as "call-outs" extending from parts to be identified to the identifying label. Commercial letters on white block background can be glued to the suitcase. Add hinges, latches, and handle.

3. Suitcases for temporary exhibits can be made by mounting four different surfaces on the inside and outside. Consider light-weight sheet metal for magnetic display; pegboard, cork, Cellotex, or Hook n' Loop®. Neither flannel nor felt is suitable, as objects will not adhere to the vertical surfaces. Add hinges, latches, and handle.

This is another type of aid that is most useful when there is no permanent classroom, as a station in a Learning Center, for individual study or for small group work.

Slides. 35mm. slides can add another dimension to the materials brought into the classroom. If desired, a taped script can be prepared to accompany the slides.

Creative facilitators can think of many situations which will lend themselves to being illustrated by slides. To cite but a few examples:

1. When a field trip is impractical or when one wishes to have a visual record for long-term use.

    A. Community problems
        1. Air and/or water pollution
        2. Sanitation
        3. Safety hazards
        4. Housing
        5. Littering
        6. Vandalism
    B. School problems
        1. Vandalism
        2. Safety hazards
        3. Overcrowding
        4. Littering

C. Community services and programs
   1. Sewage treatment
   2. Health Department
   3. Voluntary Health Agencies
   4. Water treatment
2. When it is necessary to get candid shots or set up contrived situations.
   A. Grooming patterns
   B. Conduct and manners. Common occurrences can be taken. Situations can be staged and photographed.
3. When illustrations that would be useful are found in magazines or books which are not available in quantity or from which they must not be removed.
4. To keep a record of students' projects or bulletin boards. These can be used with future classes as sources of ideas they might like to duplicate. Bulletin board slides can be analyzed for effectiveness and as sources for ideas for color combinations.

Some schools have photography classes or clubs. The teacher or advisor is a good source of information if one is not familiar with photographic techniques. The most difficult task is taking pictures of illustrations.

Assuming that an ectographic visual maker is not available, a single-lens reflex camera is the easiest to work with. Replace the lens with a macro (copy) lens. Mount the camera on a stand and place the copy flat on a table. Cover the unwanted area with white paper. Focus the camera and use an artificial light supply if necessary. Have the film processed. Any undesired area that shows on the finished slides can be blocked out by masking tape. Label the frame with the source or the name of the student who made the project.

Again, students may be involved. It is not uncommon for a student to have his own camera and be interested in photography. Frequently students will be more knowledgeable about photography than is the facilitator. Learn from them! Such students may be interested in taking a series of photos as a project. Copies can be made inexpensively to add to the departmental files.

Students can view the slides as an entire class, individually, or in small groups. Previously made sets of slides may also be previewed by students to judge whether they can be useful to illustrate an individual or group report.

Filmstrips. There are many excellent commercial filmstrips. Most of the better ones are in kit form and include a disc recording or a cassette tape containing an audio script.

Student committees can preview preselected filmstrips to choose the one they judge to be of most value for their class. Their judgment tends to be more in tune with that of their peers than is the facilitator's. It is extremely important that the filmstrips be preselected by the facilitator. Students rarely will be able to judge the accuracy of the "facts" presented. One cannot assume that the producers are presenting unbiased, factually accurate information. They may be "cashing-in" on the demand for certain topical material.

The facilitator can prepare an evaluation form that covers the information desired. Table 5 is a sample of such a form. Serving on preview committees can assist students in becoming more critical of the audiovisual materials to which they are exposed both in school and out.

TABLE 5

FILMSTRIP PREVIEW FORM

Title:...B/W or color:....................No. Frames:............
Recording: (yes)   (no)

	Yes	No	Questionable
1. Will the filmstrip help in achieving the behavioral objectives?			
2. Is the script realistic?			
3. Is the quality of the audio good?			
4. Is the quality of the visual good?			
5. Could the situations portrayed lead to good class discussions?			
6. Does it present factual information that we should know?			
7. Do you recommend that this filmstrip be shown to the class?			
Comments:			

Rank the filmstrip previewed from best (1) to poorest (3).

Preview Committee:

....

....

....

Class Day/Time ....

Films. The 16 mm. film can use techniques that are not possible in filmstrips. Through motion, the producer can present dramatizations, flashbacks, animated action, actual occurrences, discussions, interviews, and microscopic action. The combination of motion and sound tends to elicit some type of emotional response in the viewer.

It is extremely important that films be previewed. Inappropriate films are thus eliminated before students see them. When a desirable film has been selected, the facilitator has time to plan appropriate follow-up activities that will involve students.

Unfortunately many teachers find the previewing of films an impossible and unrealistic task. Films often must be ordered in the spring for the following year. Teachers that attend professional conventions have the opportunity to preview the newer films. When the films are not available, however, choices are made on the basis of film catalog write-ups or recommendations from colleagues. With a flexible program, it is extremely difficult to predict in the spring the date in the following winter when one is going to want a film.

When a school system has its own film library, the problem is compounded by requests from several teachers for the same films during the same time period. With an in-system delivery service, the chances are remote that a facilitator will receive a film on the desired date. Receiving it in time to preview it is an even more remote possibility.

Facilitators who are able to rent films from outside sources have the best opportunity for preview. Even here, what frequently occurs is that the film is "previewed" with the first class. Planning is quickly and superficially done. Revisions are made for each successive class during the next showing of the film.

These conditions make it impractical to involve students in previewing films. There is an opportunity, however, for students to comment after having seen the film. Based on their reaction and his own, the facilitator may eliminate the film from the following year's order.

A facilitator will find it helpful to keep a film file, by topic, of those films well received by students. As new films become available or as opportunities arise for previewing, they too can be filed. This makes the ordering of films a routine detail.

In addition to school and rental sources, one should survey the local sources for free films. Check the local library, the governmental health agencies, as well as the voluntary health agencies.

When planning the use of a film, it is recommended that the facilitator avoid merely "rehashing" the film content that focuses on the film characters. Instead, put your students "in the scene." Focus on them! This involves developing "iffy" questions—e.g., "What would you do if you were in Paul's position?" "If you were faced with this situation, what would you do?" Table 6 on page 124 gives a suggested guidesheet for planning film usage.

TABLE 6

GUIDESHEET FOR FILM USAGE

1. Film Title:... Time:.......................
2. Color: .... Black and White: ....
3. Concept:
4. For what purpose could the film be useful? Introduce a concept............
   Clarify a concept............. Summarize a concept..............
5. What general behavioral objectives would be applicable?
6. On which domain and in which dimension are you focusing?
7. What specific behavioral objective that utilizes the above domain and
   dimension are you using for this plan?
8. State your *planned* introduction:
9. Follow-up plan for remainder of class period. (Actively involve students by (1) putting them in the situations portrayed or (2) encouraging them to apply the concepts to their lives.)

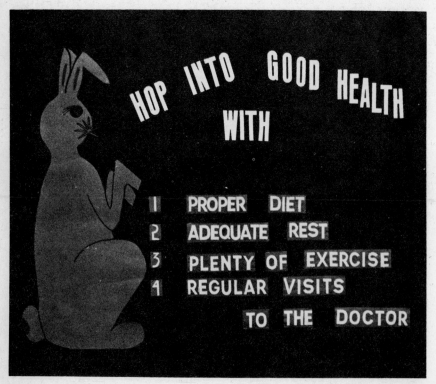

— Mary Ann King, Kent State University

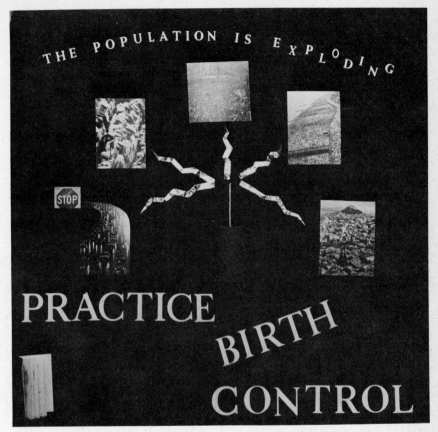

THE POPULATION IS EXPLODING

PRACTICE BIRTH CONTROL

— Ginger Hendricks, Kent State University

Videotape Recorder. Facilitators have developed ingenious ways of utilizing the videotape recorder (VTR) to enhance the learning experiences. Basically, the VTR is a portable unit consisting of a motion picture camera connected to a tape recorder with a self-contained monitor screen. Classroom activities or other programs can be recorded on the tape and replayed at a later time. The tapes may be filed or, when no longer needed, erased and the tape reused.

Some schools will have a television expert. In this case, the facilitator requisitions the unit, and an operator is assigned to do the filming. In other schools, a paraprofessional has the responsibility for setting up the equipment and the teacher does the taping. Teachers are trained to use the equipment during in-service programs. Again, the use made of the unit is dependent upon the creativity of the facilitator. As usual, the suggestions that follow are not meant to be all-inclusive.

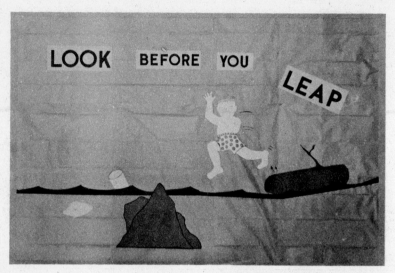

— Kathy Smoltz, Kent State University

1. *Large group presentations.* These may be pretaped or done "live" in
    one class and replayed for successive classes. The great advantage of
    this procedure is to save the facilitator from presenting the lecture
    repeatedly. All students thus receive the same information. Also,
    the tapes may be placed in the Learning Center, library, or audio-
    visual room and made available to students who missed the large
    group class.

    Through creative and imaginative thinking, the health education facil-
itator can make television lessons more than just a rehash of old and tried
classroom methods. But the preprofessional must be aware that everything done before the camera must be carefully planned and prepared.
One way in which he might familiarize himself with the use of television is
to prepare a health education lesson, complete with behavioral objectives
and audio visual aids, and record it on videotape. He might then pre-
evaluate his presentation. This would allow the preprofessional to have a
student's-eye view of himself. With the use of the tape, he could focus
on particular aspects of the teaching-learning process and study them re-
peatedly to determine strengths as well as weaknesses.

2. *Demonstrations.* The facilitator can televise effective demonstrations
    or experiments to his entire body of students. This can be done "on
    the spot" or on videotape. Television makes this method even better
    because of its effectiveness as an audio visual device. Objects that
    are too tiny, too intricate, too costly, too rare, or too dangerous to
    actually have on hand and show can be shown on television so that

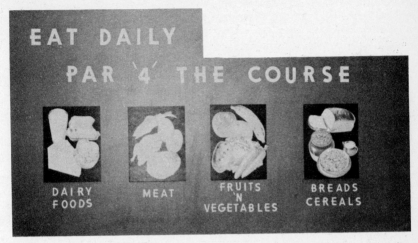

EAT DAILY

PAR '4' THE COURSE

DAIRY FOODS   MEAT   FRUITS N VEGETABLES   BREADS CEREALS

— Michaela Richards, Kent State University

every student has a front row seat. In addition, TV can magnify book pages, microscopic slides, charts and pictures because of the close-up mobility of the entire camera or the use of the zoom lens.

3. *Student presentations.* One advantage that television has for these presentations is that they need only be done once and those students giving them need not miss other classes. Such student-involving activities as panel discussions, socio dramas, skits, project presentations, interviews, oral reports, and survey results lend themselves well to television. The best of these may then be selected and presented in a large group to all health students. The students themselves, with instruction, may even participate in the actual televising.

4. *Assemblies.* Very often health education facilitators are fortunate in having available the services of an outside speaker who carries a message of importance to the total school population. The facilitator may choose to present the speaker in an assembly program to all health education students and televise the message to all other students throughout the school.

5. *Field trips.* The advent of the shoulder "pack-type" videotape recorder equipment now makes it possible to record highlights of significant field trips for later use.

6. *Educational television station programs.* Frequently educational television stations have excellent programs dealing with vital health issues. A contractual agreement can be made between the school and the station to reproduce any program in the station library. When there

is to be a program relevant to a specific concept, the facilitator may arrange with the Audio visual Department of his school to have this program taped. A timer is set to turn on the VTR at the pre-arranged time, which is frequently during the night after the station is off the air. The taped program can then be used as desired by the facilitator.

7. *Self-Instruction.* Techniques can be devised by the facilitator to allow the student to learn by self-instruction from tapes of lectures, demonstrations, experiments, or pre- and post-testing. This method may be a part of a directed study packet and is similar to that used with computerized instruction described in chapter 5, page 68.

8. *Aid to team teaching.* A teacher with a background in a specific area could present this area to all classes through television. If video-taped this could better prepare other team members for the learning activities to follow.

8

THE REALITY OF ARRIVING

In this age of accountability the facilitator is faced with the reality of proving that he has, in fact, arrived. No longer can a teacher travel along in his career and think smugly to himself, "I don't know exactly where I am going, but I'm making darn good time!" The facilitator and student of today *must* know what their destination is (goals and objectives), how they are going to arrive there (learning activities), and finally whether the trip was worthwhile (evaluation). More and more the public is demanding learning results from its monumental investment. More and more the individual facilitator or facilitating team is feeling the pressure of demonstrating or measuring these results. The success of facilitating is directly related to the proper evaluation.

Evaluation is simply a measurement of student learning and teacher effectiveness. It indicates the direction learning is going. If the evaluation is properly made and utilized, the facilitator can determine whether learning *is* taking place and whether that learning is in the direction of the designed concepts and objectives planned in advance.

The results of evaluating can also be used in future planning by the facilitator. If the results are nebulous or indecisive, he will know that he must revise his planning or evaluative techniques, or both.

In the traditional school the evaluation of student performance is almost entirely a teacher-planned and teacher-executed judgment. Today schools are seeing evaluation as a cooperative effort involving the facilitator (or team) and the student. Whereas the traditional teacher depends heavily upon questions and answers in oral recitation or the objective or subjective written-type tests, the facilitator of learning sees the student participating in the judgment of his own performance, that of his fellow student, and even that of the facilitator.

The major problem in evaluating the behaviors stated in the health education objectives is that one cannot measure long-term goals. It is impossible to evaluate health behaviors that will occur when the student is away from the influence of the classroom situation. The hope of the facilitator, then, is that he will be able to offer his students such relevant and meaningful learning experiences within the bounds of his influence that they will choose to exhibit some of these behaviors beyond the classroom.

The task of evaluating in health education, of necessity, must remain within the limitations of the classroom. The opportunity for using a variety of evaluating techniques is, however, unlimited. As the preprofessional begins to think conceptually and develops skill in the writing of behavioral objectives, he will soon discover that the door is wide open for evaluating beyond the confines of the cognitive domain. He will realize that all behavioral objectives are not stated in terms of knowledge, but that they may be written as easily in terms of the *application* of knowledge. Thus the evaluation may be tailored in keeping with the affective and psychomotor domains as well. This is not to say that the cognitive-type evaluation techniques should not be used. It is obvious that one must measure knowledge. An advantage of the objective and subjective types of testing is that they are a precise measurement of facts. But the scope of measuring goes beyond the simple recall of knowledge. In health education there are other commodities, such as attitudes, feelings, values, and skills, that should be evaluated.

If a student can learn to *apply* a concept, then it is apparent that he *knows* it. "Application" is the key word. A simple example of a health behavior that almost all students are aware of is washing the hands before eating. They *know* it should be done and yet, through experience, they have learned that usually nothing drastic happens when they have skipped this practice occasionally. As a result, if it is convenient, they will wash their hands. If it isn't, they won't. The knowledge is there, the application is not. If given opportunities to apply health knowledge to structured situations or projects within the health education class, the students become familiarized with the values of application. If a health behavior becomes important to them, in spite of all the conditions that influence their lives, they will apply it. It is the degree of importance that they attach to a behavior that will determine whether they practice it. The facilitator's responsibility, then, is to present health-learning opportunities. He *cannot* or *should not* be able to control the application of these knowledges.

All preprofessionals are familiar with ordinary cognitive-type evaluation techniques, such as the objective and subjective tests. They have experienced these through the years of their educational experience. This chapter will not include these in the discussion of evaluative methods. It is suggested that the preprofessional, if he wishes to make a comprehensive study of these types of testing, should avail himself of a course in tests and measurements.

The purpose of this book is not to philosophize on evaluation, but rather to suggest some evaluative techniques that the facilitator might consider using. In keeping with the ideology of the book, however, the authors also aim at stressing the participation of the student in the planning, the learning, and the judgment of learning performance in himself and others.

Along with these suggestions the preprofessional health educator will detect another challenge (you've had a few) by the authors—that he ought to think in terms of developing a sophisticated attitude toward evaluation. Perhaps, even, this attitude should be one of de-emphasizing the grade and emphasizing the total development of the student. Too often objective testing takes place under conditions of pressure and emotion that result in "learning for the moment." If a student fails, it is likely that he will "turn off." Every youngster should be given every opportunity to succeed. Failure, which may be a way of life for some students, need not be reinforced in health education. The evaluation of a student's performance should include not only the knowledge he accumulates, but also the development of his total personality. Perhaps, if a student fails, the teacher has failed to come up with an evaluative procedure adequate for measuring the total learning the student has experienced.

Evaluation should, then, measure behavioral changes that occur in a student as a result of learning. It is toward this end that the balance of the chapter will be devoted. To be discussed are teacher-contrived evaluations, student self-evaluations, student evaluation of students, student evaluation of facilitator performance, and facilitator self-evaluation.

Teacher-Contrived Evaluation

Evaluation in the classroom is an ongoing process. A facilitator is constantly evaluating his students in one way or another, structured or unstructured. A fact of life that he must accept is that not all students are going to learn everything, no matter how great the facilitator envisions himself. Total effectiveness is an aim but not a goal. He may expect that much learning will take place. Conversely he may expect that much will not. The sooner the facilitator becomes comfortable with this knowledge, the better off he will be. He must remain flexible and vary his methods of measuring learning so as best to offer opportunities for success to his students.

Teacher—Question. A variety of tools may be used by the facilitator to help him arrive at a fair evaluation of learning. One of these is the "teacher-question."[3] The preprofessional should become familiar with

3. Adapted from "Teacher Questions," Berea (Ohio) School System. Used with permission.

categories of teacher questions. Each substantive teacher-question can be categorized in terms of the effect it is likely to have in stimulating cognitive or affective behavior on the part of the students involved. The system to be scrutinized by the preprofessional in categorizing teacher-questions is as follows:

Cognitive Domain

1. Recognition—Question asks for simple choices: Which of these? Was it this way or that? Is it true or false?
2. Recall—Question asks for recall of specific information: Who was it? What is the answer? Can you recall what it was?
3. Demonstration of skill—Question asks for skill to be shown in use: Can you show us? Can you trace the flow on the transparency?
4. Comprehension—Question asks for information showing simple relationships: Can you give me an example? What do you mean?
5. Analysis—Question asks for information organized to reveal cause-and-effect relationships or complete inter-relationships: Why did this happen? Can you describe similarities and differences?
6. Synthesis—Question asks for use of information to form new generalizations or draw conclusions or inferences: What principle can you see in this? What would happen if . . .? How could this problem be approached? How would you evaluate the decision?

Affective Domain

7. Opinion—Question asks for expression of simple opinion: What do you suppose? How would you feel? What would you do? What do you think should be done?
8. Attitude or Value—Question asks for expressions of complex feelings or attitudes: Why do you *feel* this way? Can you tell us how you feel? From your point of view, what issues are involved?

Many ways can be listed here to accomplish teacher evaluation of the individual student or the groups in which he operates. But in the long run the facilitator will create his own techniques to reach the objectives as he has prescribed them. Since most preprofessionals have been inundated with methods that measured only knowledge, the challenge of creativity again looms before him.

Casting aside those familiar types of teacher testing (essay, true-false, multiple choice, completion, and matching) we see other means to reach the desired objectives.

Open-Ended Sentences. This type of evaluation not only allows the student considerable freedom, but can also indicate to the facilitator some of the applicable knowledge the student has accumulated. Open-ended sentences can be used to evaluate in either the cognitive or affective domain, or both. When using this technique, the facilitator must assure the student that he will not be graded on his opinions. Rather than a grade as such, the facilitator will be able to gain insight into a student's attitudes, values, and beliefs. A few examples of open-ended sentences in health education are the following:

1. In regard to sex education, all parents should . . .
2. If I needed to lose ten pounds, I would probably . . .
3. If I needed a pain killer, I would . . .
4. Environmental conditions within our school would be improved if . . .
5. When I don't feel well, I . . .
6. If I knew someone was pushing drugs, I would . . .
7. My personal responsibilities toward world health are . . .
8. My reasons for (eating) (not eating) breakfast are . . .

Position Paper. Another suggested teacher-structured evaluative technique is the position paper.

Directions: Take a position on the following controversial issue.
Resolved: The use of marijuana should be legalized in the United States.

I do/do not support this resolution. (CIRCLE ONE)

From what sources would you gather enough information to convince me that your answer is right? Be specific. State each resource and give a brief quotation from it that you feel is important. One point will be awarded for each valid resource used. If you find more than ten different sources that support your position, you will receive an "A"; seven to nine, a "B"; three to six, a "C"; one or two, a "D."

All available materials from the school and the health education libraries are available on the table at the front of the room. You may use any others you can find on your own, such as newspaper articles. Sooner or later you may, in your daily life, actually be asked to face this issue.

Health/Art Project. The psychomotor domain also may be incorporated in conjunction with either of the other domains or both. The following is a suggested method that the facilitator might consider:

Directions: Read carefully. We have been discovering the importance of proper nutrition in our total living. Choose one of the following ways to express the need to include all four of the basic food groups in our daily diet:

1. Mobile
2. Collage
3. Cartoon
4. Papier-mâché sculpture

This assignment is to be done at home with any materials you can find. Be original! Be colorful! Say something in your project! Be neat! Your grade will be judged on a basis of four points for outstanding; three points for very good; two points for good; and one point for fair in each of these categories:

—————— ORIGINALITY
—————— COLORFULNESS
—————— CLARITY OF MESSAGE
—————— NEATNESS OF FINISHED PROJECT

Together we will determine the grading scale—how many points will make an A—B—C—D?

The preprofessional will see here that this type of assignment not only can be judged by the facilitator, but can be used also as a student self-evaluator or means for evaluation by other students.

Student Self-Appraisal

As mentioned earlier, the emphasis of this book is on involvement by the student in his total learning experience. When he is given full consideration in the planning of his learning and in the setting up of the criteria for his own evaluation, the entire process becomes more meaningful to him. This is not to say that the student will immediately begin to learn more or that discipline problems will cease to exist. But in the kinds of learning described in this text neither the teacher nor the student is necessarily "on stage." Learning is a team effort and both are working together to reach the objectives. The possibility for the student to move from less desirable to more desirable behaviors does exist. Not to be ignored is the fact that the facilitator is experiencing learning at the same time.

By the very nature of its content health education must begin to emphasize learning in the affective domain. The same "hang-up" exists in our area as in any other discipline that stresses valuing. That "block" to many facilitators is in evaluation. This is an unnecessary frustration. There are many ways that the facilitator will discover, as he moves along, for planning affective learnings, for getting his students involved, and for developing valid criteria by which to judge performance. Remember that the best methods for evaluation to meet the needs of each individual situation are the self-discovered ones.

First, let us suggest that sometime at the beginning of the school year, the facilitator devote an entire class session to discussing grades with the students. Let them develop the criteria on the basis of which they will be graded, and by whom. If they know that they are setting up their own evaluation basis, they will certainly know what their responsibilities are. Perhaps, with their suggestions in mind, the facilitator will then be able to come up with an evaluation form similar to the following by which a student can judge his own performance.

Student Progress Report. *Directions:* Read carefully. Rate your own progress in this health education concept thus far for each of the following items. If you feel that your contribution has been outstanding, give yourself a grade of 5; if it was good, assign a 4; if you feel your performance was so-so, give yourself a 3; if barely acceptable, mark a 2; if you "bombed," enter a 1. (Everyone "bombs" in some phase sometime.)

.... 1.   Your contribution to the total class (or small group).

.... 2.   The interest and ambition you have demonstrated in this concept.

.... 3.   How much learning growth you achieved in this concept.

.... 4.   Is your small group better off for your having been there?

.... 5.   Have you communicated with others?

.... 6.   How well you pulled your fair share of the load.

.... 7.   Offered ideas or thoughts that others could build upon.

.... 8.   Stuck to the task and tried to do the job that had to be done.

.... 9.   Contributed extra effort to ensure the success of the group in meeting its responsibility.

........10.   Did extra (unassigned) reading in the concept.

........11.   To what extent did you become personally involved?

........12.   How open to others' suggestions, ideas, and values were you?

........TOTAL SCORE (POSSIBLE 60 PTS.)

At the end of a concept or about one week before the grading period ends, the facilitator should have each student fill out his own evaluation report and hand it in. He should then have the class decide on what they think the grading scale should be. Finally, with the self-evaluation in hand, he may have a short one-to-one interview with each student concerning the criteria and his self-rating. Surprisingly enough, the facilitator will probably discover that students evaluate themselves fairly honestly. If they do not, their peers will soon set them straight.

Self-Appraisal In Understanding a Concept. The facilitator may wish to have the student appraise his own understanding of particular behavioral objectives. This may be done in the following suggested manner. Please note that this suggestion is being presented in a generalized form. The verbs in the evaluative statement may be any of those indicated in the behavioral objective.

CONCEPT DESCRIPTION ....

NAME .... DATE ....

Directions: As a final check, rate yourself on the objectives of this concept. For each, use the five-point scale indicated:

(1)	(2)	(3)	(4)	(5)
Yes, very much				No, very little

After having completed this concept, I am able to:

........1. Identify (add specific content according to concept)

........2. Recognize ....

........3. Trace ....

........4. List ....

........5. Explain ....

Place any comments you have on the back of this sheet.

If you have rated yourself a 4 or 5 on any of the objectives, you may wish to contact me privately for additional help or clarification. It is *not* a sign of weakness to ask for help. We all learn by asking questions.

Grading Period Self-Appraisal. At the end of the grading periods the facilitator may even choose to involve the student in the determination of his final grades. This could be accomplished in a way similar to the following:

NAME: ....

DATE: ....

NINE WEEKS GRADE ....

Directions: Rate yourself on each of the following statements. Use a 5-point scale. If the statement describes you very well, use a 5. If it does not fit you at all, use a 1.

........1. I always make constructive use of my time in class.

........2. I participate in class activities and ask questions when I do not understand.

........3. My attendance is good and I am always on time for class.

........4. I come to class everyday prepared to work.

........5. When necessary, I spend enough time outside the classroom on assignments to guarantee my understanding of the material.

........6. I have tried not to distract my fellow students from their learning.

........7. I feel I have a good understanding of the concepts studied during this grading period.

........8. I really believe that I have done the best that I am capable of.

In view of your evaluation of yourself, what letter grade do you think you should receive for this grading period?

Comments:

Student Evaluation of Students

The value of student appraisal of fellow students is yet to be discovered by most present-day teachers. Up to this time the entire evaluative process has been almost entirely retained as a cherished function of the teacher, and the teacher solely. This has been his domain, and he has reigned over the flock with absolute authority. The grade that he judged to be accurate was his reward to his students for a job performed or not performed according to the standards that he set forth. Very rarely did the thought of evaluation as a cooperative effort enter into his thinking. Even today, as education is undergoing a great metamorphosis, many teachers are remaining motionless, especially in the area of evaluation. The thought of students judging each other's learning will be considered highly questionable or be summarily dismissed by them. This area will be held sacrosanct by the traditionalists.

Again the preprofessional will hear the cry of "challenge!" that he has so many times encountered in the pages of this book. Who is to say that many heads are not better than one, even if they are students' heads? On the same plane, isn't their judgment valid since they are evaluating learning from their point of view? Certainly their thinking is relevant to them. They are aware of learning that is meaningful to them. Even if their judgments and thoughts may not totally coincide with those of the facilitator, the evaluative basis is widened when the students are given the opportunity to evaluate one another. This technique should be considered by the preprofessional.

Student evaluation of other students may be done by an individual student or by group consensus. The facilitator can decide which. He may want to vary the format to fit the circumstances.

Many methods of learning lend themselves well to student evaluations of one another. Some that do are sociodramas, skits, projects, bulletin boards, oral reports, panel discussions, and small group discussions. *One important point must be made here.* Criteria must be developed by which the student evaluates the performance of another. These criteria are dependent upon the learning activity and should be tailored for that particular purpose. Again, the students may or may not be involved in the designing of the criteria. The criteria should be as objective as possible so that a degree of reliability may be assured.

With the thought in mind that he will better be able to formulate his own evaluative tools to suit his particular needs, the preprofessional is asked to consider the following suggestions. Remember that the facilitator, as well as the student, may use the same criteria for judgment.

Bulletin Board Evaluation. *Directions:* Please evaluate the bulletin board by placing a check for each item in the column you deem appropriate.

Location of board .... Title .... Date ....

CRITERIA	OUTSTANDING	EXCELLENT	GOOD	AVERAGE	FAIR	POOR
1. Is factually accurate.						
2. Has a message.						
3. Shows originality and creativity.						
4. Has eye appeal.						
5. Good use of color/color contrast.						
6. Has a focal point.						
7. Can be seen from a distance.						
8. Makes good use of space (design).						
9. Is appropriate for audience served.						
10. Display neatly constructed.						
11. Has a border.						
12. Lettering clear and correct.						
13. Labeling grammatically correct.						

Additional comments:

Small Group Discussion Evaluation.[1] (Forced Choice Evaluation of Individual's Contributions.)

Directions: By his very presence each member of the group made a contribution to the solving of the problem. There are roles that are helpful and roles that are destructive in achieving the group task. To help you, some of these are listed below:

Helpful: Initiates action, is friendly, considerate of others' ideas, a good listener, praises others, keeps the group on the track, summarizes, carries his share of the load, is constructive, gives reasons for his opinion, is helpful, evaluates ideas objectively, is factual, reduces group tension with humor, facilitates participation by others.

Destructive: Refuses to participate, "turns off" ideas of others, tries to block discussion, "needles" others without reason, could not care less about the group and its task, tries to force group to go in his direction,

1. Courtesy of Dr. Virginia Harvey, Professor, Counselor and Personnel Services Education, Kent State University, Kent, Ohio. By permission.

is impolite, rejects the rights of others, wanders aimlessly off the track, fails to listen to other opinions, avoids carrying his share of the load, demonstrates disruptive behavior.

Visualize a continuum. Where would you place each member of your group on it? Place each individual's name on the line in the order you feel is right.

<table>
<tr><td>Eggbert</td><td>Isaac</td></tr>
<tr><td>EFFECTIVE</td><td>INEFFECTIVE</td></tr>
</table>

List each individual in your group, including yourself, in the order of his helpfulness to the group on accomplishing the task. Give your reasons for the ranking.

This is a "forced-choice" item. No two people may receive the same ranking.

Name	Reasons
1.	
2.	
3.	
4.	
5.	
6.	

Student Reaction to Small Group Experience[2]

NAME .... DATE ....

Directions: Please evaluate your small group by answering the following questions in the manner designated.

1. How worthwhile was this learning experience to you?

........Very worthwhile ....Fairly worthwhile ....Somewhat worthwhile ....Fairly unworthwhile ....Very unworthwhile

2. I feel (check at the appropriate point on scale) about the way our group worked.

Highly satisfied ____5____4____3____2____1____ Highly dissatisfied

2. *Ibid.*

3. I am (check the scale) with the decisions we made.
Highly satisfied _____ 5   4   3   2   1 _____ Highly dissatisfied
4. To what degree were members open and leveling with each other about their thoughts, feelings and attitudes?
Great deal _____ 5   4   3   2   1 _____ Practically not at all
5. What did you feel were the strong points of your small group?
6. What do you feel were the weak points of your small group?
7. Any additional comments you wish to make about this learning experience:

Sociodrama Evaluation

TITLE OF SOCIODRAMA ....

DATE ....

Directions: Please evaluate the socio drama presented by placing a check in the column you feel is appropriate for each statement.

Evaluative Statement	Agree	Disagree
1. Situation was realistically portrayed.		
2. Players approached roles seriously.		
3. Held interest of audience.		
4. Voices carried well.		
5. Socio drama demonstrated the behavior exhibited in the objective.		
6. Set stage well for follow-up discussion.		

7. COMMENTS OR SUGGESTIONS:

                                        NAMES

....
....
....
....

Panel Discussion Evaluation

SUBJECT OF DISCUSSION ....
NAMES:

                ....
                ....
                ....

DATE ....

CLASS PERIOD:..

Directions: Using the scale below as a guide, please evaluate the panel discussion by placing the number you consider appropriate in the left-hand column preceding each of the statements.

4	3	2	1
Strongly agree	Agree	Disagree	Strongly disagree

NUMBER	STATEMENT
.... 1.	Panel was well prepared.
.... 2.	Presentation was well organized.
.... 3.	Cited sources of factual information.
.... 4.	Held attention of audience.
.... 5.	Maintained eye contact with audience.
.... 6.	Used visual aids to clarify.
.... 7.	Infrequent dependence on notes.
.... 8.	Stayed on subject.
.... 9.	All participated.
........10.	Used good English.
........11.	Valuable information given.
....	TOTAL POINTS

Other comments:

Skit Evaluation

TITLE OF SKIT ....

NAMES:

....

....

....

DATE ....

CLASS PERIOD:..

Directions: Please evaluate the skit presented by circling either "yes" or "no" following each evaluative statement.

1. Showed planning and forethought. (Yes—No)
2. Demonstrated originality and creativity. (Yes—No)
3. Used effective props. (Yes—No)
4. Roles were realistically portrayed. (Yes—No)
5. Held interest of audience. (Yes—No)
6. Voices carried well. (Yes—No)
7. Skit achieved its objective well. (Yes—No)
8. Set stage for follow-up discussion. (Yes—No)

Additional Comments:

Project Evaluation

PROJECT DESCRIPTION ....

NAME............................ CLASS PERIOD............... DATE.....................

Directions: Evaluate both the project and the presentation of it. For each, use the following five-point scale.

(1)	(2)	(3)	(4)	(5)
Yes, very much				No, very little

I. PROJECT
........1. Showed originality and creativity.
........2. Demonstrated quality.
........3. Achieved objective.
........4. Motivated learning.
........5. Is useful.

II. PRESENTATION
........1. Project clearly explained.
........2. Presented so all could see.
........3. Voice could be heard.
........4. Competently used equipment needed.
........5. Maintained eye contact with audience.
........6. Accomplished the objective.

Additional comments:

Oral Report Evaluation

Directions: Evaluate the speaker and the report by circling the number you feel is appropriate.

NAME: .... TOPIC: .... DATE: ....

1. Demonstrated preparation and planning.

(0)	(1)	(2)
No	Most of the time	Yes

2. Presented topic well.

(0)	(1)	(2)
No	Most of the time	Yes

3. Held interest of audience.

(0)	(1)	(2)
No	Most of the time	Yes

4.   Speaker free from annoying mannerisms.

(0)	(1)	(2)
No	Most of the time	Yes

5.   Voice could be heard.

(0)	(1)	(2)
No	Most of the time	Yes

6.   Little dependence on notes.

(0)	(1)	(2)
No	Most of the time	Yes

7.   Good use of English.

(0)	(1)	(2)
No	Most of the time	Yes

8.   Maintained eye contact.

(0)	(1)	(2)
No	Most of the time	Yes

9.   Report contributed to the understanding of the concept.

(0)	(1)	(2)
No	Most of the time	Yes

Additional comments:

Student Evaluation of Facilitator

Some facilitators may be very hesitant about allowing their students to evaluate their performance as a facilitator of learning. They may feel that this is a threat to them, whether they admit it or not. They may rationalize why they choose *not* to include this measurement of themselves— "My students are too immature to judge me." "What do they know about teaching?" "This is going too far with evaluation—after all, I am the teacher, they are the students." "The kids in my classes would welcome a chance to 'shoot me down.'" "Our school is too traditional to accept this." "What good would it do, anyway?" "I don't think I could trust my kids to do this." "The kids of today already have too much freedom in education." "Maybe the truth will hurt."

You could probably list many more of these types of rationalizations that teachers might use for not allowing students to evaluate them as facilitators. However, examine those mentioned above. The preprofessional might ask himself, "How do *I* know these rationalizations amount to valid reasons if I never allow the students to evaluate me?"

If the facilitator gives much thought and planning to the ways *he evaluates his students and their learning,* why would it not be fair to allow the students a chance to evaluate objectively his success in facilitating learning? Examine once again the enumeration of reasons why not. Can you, as a preprofessional, detect that many of these reasons might be symptoms of teacher inadequacy? There may be reasons why kids *would* welcome a chance to "shoot down" a teacher, personally or professionally. There may be reasons *why* a teacher would feel threatened.

Accountability is a two-way street. While it is important to evaluate the achievement of students, it is equally important and desirable to evaluate the achievement of facilitators. Evaluation *by students* might enlighten any facilitator as to his particular strengths or weaknesses. As a result, with mutual trust, the learning experiences of both the students and the facilitator might be more easily expedited.

The bold preprofessional will view student evaluation of facilitating as a means of professional growth. In this competitive world he should seize every opportunity for strengthening his effectiveness in reaching his students and facilitating learning.

Evaluation of Facilitator Performance

Consider the following example of a student-evaluation of the facilitator:

Directions: We have just finished this phase of our learning. In order to improve his/her competence, your teacher is asking you to fill out the following evaluation of his teaching performance in this concept. You need not sign your name. Please mark each item.

	Very good	Good	Fair	Poor
1. Knowledge of subject matter.				
2. Evidence of planning.				
3. Subject interestingly presented.				
4. Student involvement sought in learning activities and evaluations.				
5. Teacher guidance in learning.				
6. Rapport with students.				
7. Class morale.				
8. Classroom management.				
9. Voice.				
10. Vitality.				
11. Appearance.				
12. My overall evaluation of the way this concept was presented.				

13. Other comments:

The facilitator might wish to use an evaluation of the total health education program for the year, by the students. This could prove to be very valuable in pointing out what they consider to be:

1. The more meaningful (to them) content areas;
2. The overall effectiveness of the teaching;
3. The methods of learning used they enjoyed most; and
4. The changes in content or methods they feel should be made.

The results of such an evaluation may prove invaluable in future planning.

The preprofessional should think about the following suggested evaluation tools, but he should remember that, more than likely, he will come up with some which will better meet his own needs.

Evaluation of the Health Education Course. *Directions:* Please evaluate the health education program for this year by circling the number you consider to be suitable. You need not sign your name.

No. 1—Signifies that you strongly disagree with statement.
No. 2—Signifies that you disagree with statement.
No. 3—Indicates that you agree with statement.
No. 4—Indicates that you strongly agree with statement.

	1	2	3	4
I. GENERAL EVALUATION				
1. This health education experience was valuable to me.	1	2	3	4
2. The class morale seemed to be high.	1	2	3	4
3. The classroom environment was pleasant.	1	2	3	4
4. The concepts studied were relevant and meaningful to me.	1	2	3	4
5. I became involved in my health education.	1	2	3	4
6. My values in some areas were influenced by this class.	1	2	3	4
7. Most of the time I felt free to express myself.	1	2	3	4
8. The teacher and/or teaching team seemed to know their subject matter.	1	2	3	4
9. The teacher talked "with" us, not "at" us.	1	2	3	4
10. On the whole the teacher showed trust in us.	1	2	3	4
11. The teacher treated us fairly.	1	2	3	4
12. The teacher showed evidence of being well organized.	1	2	3	4
13. We had adequate resource material to refer to.	1	2	3	4

II. SPECIFIC EVALUATION
1. To me the most valuable part of the health education class this year was:
2. The least valuable part in my opinion was:
3. I feel that more time should have been spent on:
4. Less emphasis should have been put on:
5. I would suggest that the following topic be included for next year:
6. I feel that this part should be eliminated next year:
7. Additional comments:

Evaluation of Learning Activities. *Directions:* This year you have been involved in many activities designed to further your learning in health education. If you liked performing the activity, circle "Liked." If not, circle "Disliked."

1. Small group discussions. (Liked—Disliked)
2. Worksheets. (Liked—Disliked)
3. Table talk. (Liked—Disliked)
4. Panel discussions. (Liked—Disliked)
5. Health/art projects. (Liked—Disliked)
6. Bulletin board. (Liked—Disliked)
7. Sociodramas. (Liked—Disliked)
8. Oral reports on video tape. (Liked—Disliked)
9. Contests. (Liked—Disliked)
10. Original skits. (Liked—Disliked)
11. Field trip. (Liked—Disliked)
12. Movie-making. (Liked—Disliked)
13. Survey. (Liked—Disliked)
14. Interview. (Liked—Disliked)
15. Position papers. (Liked—Disliked)
16. Computer lessons. (Liked—Disliked)

Now rate these activities in the order of how you liked them. Number 1 should be the one you liked most and number 16 the one you liked least.

1.	5.	9.	13.
2.	6.	10.	14.
3.	7.	11.	15.
4.	8.	12.	16.

There are times when a facilitator may wish to have his students appraise a particular learning method after he has utilized it. This may indicate to the facilitator whether or not the method was of some value, and if so, whether to use it again, and how he might improve it. Consider the following example using "Worksheets" as the learning activity:

Appraisal of a Specific Learning Method. *Directions:* If you agree with the statement, circle the word "Agree." If you disagree, circle the word "Disagree" and explain "Why" in the space below the statement.

1. I like worksheets as a method of learning. (Agree—Disagree)

2. The questions were clearly stated. (Agree—Disagree)

3. The questions were thought-provoking. (Agree—Disagree)

4. The worksheets fit in well with the rest of the activities in this concept. (Agree—Disagree)

5. Enough time was allotted for completion. (Agree—Disagree)

6. Plenty of reference material was available. (Agree—Disagree)

7. I was encouraged to express my own opinion in answer to many questions. (Agree—Disagree)

8. The learning derived was valuable to me. (Agree—Disagree)

9. I prefer working with another student on worksheets. (Agree—Disagree)

Additional comments:

Facilitator Self-Evaluation

There is no reason why a facilitator of learning cannot grow every year in his understanding of his role. If he can unshackle his potentialities and dare now and then to take a fling at the seemingly impossible, there is only one direction he can go—forward. It is one thing to *want* to improve his craft, it is another to *do* it. So many teachers fear making mistakes or botching an effort that they build up walls of confinement from which they find it difficult to escape. The preprofessional must be mindful that mistakes, too, are valuable learning experiences, if he does something about correcting them. The recognition of an ineffective effort and its causes will enable the facilitator to advance rather than retreat in his effectuality.

If a facilitator really wants to know how things are going for him, he must be willing to take a good, hard evaluative look at his performance from time to time throughout the school year. With the changing scope and added significance of accountability, the genuinely involved facilitator will recognize the value of self-evaluation. It can aid in indicating to him whether he is accomplishing his goals with reference to student competencies as related to the objectives. Coupled with student evaluations of the facilitator, this self-appraisal may prove an invaluable aid toward self-improvement. The results may prove to be very favorable. If not, he knows the areas in which readjustment is essential.

It must be pointed out here that the authors are not proposing that at the conclusion of each concept or grading period a facilitator should make a statistical study of his effectiveness. Rather, it is suggested that he merely utilize a simple evaluative tool. Without such a reference the facilitator may well find himself perpetuating mediocre teaching patterns. It behooves him to use some kind of evaluation, whether self-contrived or otherwise. If, as was said earlier in this chapter, evaluation is an ongoing process, he must do this periodically.

The following suggested example should serve merely as a model to be implemented or changed according to the needs of the user.

Facilitator Self-Evaluation Checklist. *Directions:* Evaluate the following items by placing a check in the appropriate column.

Checklist	Yes	For the most part	No
1. I know the names of all my students.			
2. The activities were designed to involve students.			
3. Students participated in planning the objectives.			
4. Students participated in the evaluation of their learning.			
5. Content was relevant to the students' world and their problems.			
6. There was evidence that the students were motivated.			
7. Students displayed enthusiasm.			
8. I was a facilitator more than a "sage on stage."			
9. I listened more than I talked.			
10. I felt that rapport existed in the classroom.			
11. Students asked questions.			

12. Students came in for additional help.			
13. I was available to my students when needed.			
14. My resources and information were up-to-date.			
15. Students used the resources.			
16. There was evidence of student inter-action.			
17. Students showed evidence of self-discipline.			
18. When necessary to impose discipline, I was able to handle my own.			
19. I recognized and spoke to my students out of class.			
20. I felt that I was able to "reach" my students.			
21. I cooperated with other members of my teaching team.			
22. I carried my fair share of the load.			
23. I was open to suggestions.			
24. The objectives in this concept were reached.			

Conclusion

The preprofessional should consider evaluation and evaluation methods seriously. Grading, as such, is being de-emphasized. Learning is receiving the stress, and rightfully so. In keeping with this forward trend, there have been examples of evaluative techniques presented in this chapter which may trigger the thinking of the individual facilitator. The hope is, then, that he will be able to develop his own evaluative tools to meet his particular needs.

SAMPLE COMPUTER LESSONS

Cognitive Domain—No. 1

Concept: Use of the substances that modify mood and behavior arises from a variety of motivations.

Behavioral Objective: The student is able to indicate on a multiple-choice preassessment test his knowledge of mood modifiers.

Directions: Type in the *letter* of the choice that makes the following statements most correct.

1.   The introduction of "foreign" drugs into the body:

Computer Response

A.   Causes uniform effects.

The human body is in essence a chemical factory that produces drugs of its own in the form of hormones and enzymes. These substances have the function of controlling various body processes such as growth, digestion, and activity. Each person's body is different. Is there not a better answer? Try again.

B.   Often results in unexpected side-effects that can prove harmful.

You are correct. For additional information on each choice, type A; read the response; then type C; then D.

C.   Produces predictable results.

The results of taking drugs cannot be completely predictable because each person's body chemistry is different. Is there not a better answer? Try again.

D.   Has decreased our life expectancy.

Life expectancy has increased from forty-seven years in 1900 to seventy years in 1966. It is estimated that five million more Americans are alive today as a result of changes in mortality rates due to the contributions of drugs. Is there not a better answer? Try again.

2. Amphetamines serve to:

A. Stimulate the central nervous system.

You are correct. For additional information on each choice, type B; read the response; then type C; then D.

B. Calm a person down.

People under the influence of these drugs often feel capable of performing impossible and often dangerous feats; a loss of judgment. Amphetamines cause a feeling of well-being in people suffering from depression. Is there not a better answer? Try again.

C. Stimulate appetite.

Amphetamines are given as diet pills because they temporarily depress the appetite. Is there not a better answer? Try again.

D. Offer sleep to those who are nervous and have insomnia.

College students often use these pep pills to stay awake for upcoming exams. Truck drivers take them to sustain a long drive. Using them to mask fatigue is a questionable practice inasmuch as the pills are known to create a false sense of well-being and hallucinations. Is there not a better answer? Try again.

3. The use of alcohol can:

A. Be particularly damaging to the kidneys.

Though alcohol can increase urinary activity, recent studies indicate that it has no negative effect on these organs. Is there not a better answer? Try again.

B. In cases of severe intoxication, affect the liver temporarily by causing it to become enlarged and tender, resulting in symptoms of acute hepatitis.

This is correct. For additional information on each choice, type A; read the response, then type C; then D.

C. Not cause any inadequacy in nutritional status.

Prolonged heavy drinking does cause protein and Vitamin B deficiencies that hamper the ability of the liver to handle fat normally. A fatty liver is produced, which is a forerunner of cirrhosis of the liver.

D. Not cause irrita-
tion of the tissue
of the body which
comes in direct
contact with it be-
cause alcohol is
medicinal.

People who are heavy drinkers often have a chronic inflammation of the stomach lining. It can also irritate the mouth and esophagus. Anyone who has experienced the application of a strong antiseptic to a cut on the outside of the body can imagine the effects of pouring an alcoholic solution on a sore in the lining of the stomach.

4. Ever since the first report of the American Cancer Society, which linked smoking with lung cancer:

A. Cigarette manu-
facturers have
spent more money
to try to increase
sales.

Cigarette manufacturers increased advertising costs 134% from 1954 to 1961. Choice A is only a partial answer. Is there not a better answer? Try again.

B. Cigarette sales
have fluctuated.

Cigarette sales slumped to $369 billion in 1954 and increased to $490 billion in 1961. The expenditures paid off very well. In 1964 there was a significant slump due to the Surgeon-General's report. The years 1969 and 1970 show a sharp increase in sales. This is only a partial answer. Is there not a better answer? Try again.

C. The filter-tip ciga-
rette has become
more popular.

Though the filters were not very effective in filtering out tars, they did serve to satisfy the customer that he was "safe from cancer." In 1953, non-filtered cigarettes accounted for 80% of total sales. In 1963, they accounted for only 25%. Choice C is only a partial answer. Try again.

D. A, B, and C have
occurred.

You are correct. For additional information, type A; read the response, then type B; then C.

5. Chances of developing lung cancer:

A. Increase with the
number of ciga-
rettes smoked per
day.

The individual who smokes 20 cigarettes a day is ten times more likely to develop lung cancer than the nonsmoker. The 40-cigarette-a-day smoker is 21 times more likely to develop lung cancer. This is correct, but there is a better answer. Try again.

B. Increase because clinically this disease is rarely diagnosed early and of all forms is one of the most difficult to cure.

Lung cancer is often regarded as a persistent cough or cold upon which no action is taken. Choice B is only a partial answer. Is there not a better one? Try again.

C. Decrease when one smokes a pipe instead of cigarettes, provided he does not inhale.

Any individual who does not inhale minimizes the risks of developing lung cancer. Cigar smokers and pipe smokers rarely inhale. Choice C is only a partial answer. Try again.

D. Are true in A, B, and C.

You are correct. Choice D is the best answer. For additional information on each choice, type A; read the response, then type B; then C.

6. It is important to read the label on nonprescription drugs primarily:

A. Because it tells when to refill the supply and what dosage to take.

If the drugs are misused they can have serious side-effects. Since no prescription is needed, there is no control over the number of times a new supply may be purchased. Is there not a better answer? Try again.

B. Because labels give the classification of the drug.

The law requires that labels should be placed on nonprescription drugs. The label gives warnings, usage, and ingredients. The labels are very important. Is there not a better answer? Try again.

C. Because the drugs should be used only for a short period of time.

You are correct. Self-medication can be dangerous as one may have a serious condition that needs medical attention. Labels normally caution the user to see a physician if the condition persists. For additional information on each choice, type A; read the response, type B; then D.

D. Because of both A and B.

Labels refer to safe usage, when not to use, when to see a physician. Is there not a better answer? Try again.

—Sue Ledyard[1]

1. Sue Ledyard, Kent State University, Kent, Ohio. By permission

Affective Domain—No. 2

Concept: Use of substances that modify mood and behavior arises from a variety of motivations.

Behavioral Objective: The student is able to rank his feelings toward smoking marijuana.

Directions: Next to each of the following statements the student places the *letter* of the choice which best describes his attitude toward the statement.

A.   Strongly agree
B.   Agree
C.   Disagree
D.   Strongly disagree
E.   Neither agree nor disagree

.... 1.   Smoking marijuana is a way to relieve my tensions.

.... 2.   If my best friends started smoking marijuana, I probably would too.

.... 3.   I am afraid to smoke marijuana because the evidence as to its effects are inconclusive.

.... 4.   My decision whether to smoke or not is based on my own opinions rather than on other's opinions.

.... 5.   I believe smoking pot is a demonstration of rebellion against established values.

.... 6.   If I were a smoker and were asked by my coach not to smoke marijuana, I would probably quit.

.... 7.   I believe the anti-marijuana television commercials are an effective deterrent against marijuana smoking.

.... 8.   Although my parents say they would be hurt and angry if I ever smoked marijuana, I would tell them about it when I did.

.... 9.   My goals in life are to be well-adjusted, healthy, and happy. Smoking marijuana would be detrimental to these goals.

............10.   If I didn't smoke marijuana with my friends, I probably would not be accepted in my group.

............11.   Most of the reasons presented to me about why I should not smoke marijuana are reasonable and make good sense.

............12.   If smoking marijuana were not against the law, I would try it.

............13.   Smoking is just a fad which I think will be replaced by another such fad.

............14.   Others should not try to influence me against smoking marijuana because it is none of their business.

............15.   I believe everyone should try marijuana to see what it is like before making a judgment for or against it.

—Sue Ledyard[2]

2. Ibid.

Affective Domain—No. 3

Concept: Use of substances that modify mood and behavior arises from a variety of motivations.

Behavioral Objectives: The student is able to express his feelings toward statements related to smoking (tobacco) habits.

Directions: Rate each of the following statements according to the way *you* feel about it. The rating will be done on a five-point scale with:

A. Strongly agree
B. Agree
C. Neither agree nor disagree
D. Disagree
E. Strongly disagree

.... 1. My first goal is to be happy and healthy and smoking would only hinder me.
.... 2. If my parents can smoke, why can't I?
.... 3. My close friends smoke and they think it's cool.
.... 4. If I didn't smoke, I probably would not be accepted in my group.
.... 5. I would rather not smoke than be unable to play my best in athletics.
.... 6. Smoking is a way to relieve my tensions.
.... 7. I've done without smoking so far, so why should I start now?
.... 8. I clearly understand the degree to which smoking may be detrimental to my health.
.... 9. If my best friend started to smoke, I probably would also.
............10. I have heard enough about smoking to know that it is not good for me.
............11. If I were trying out for a sport and the coach told me I would have to quit smoking in order to play, I probably would quit.
............12. I was influenced to smoke by commercials that made smoking look glamorous or masculine.
............13. Anti-smoking commercials really make a lot of sense in what they say—enough to turn me away from smoking.
............14. Smoking is only a way of rebelling, so why should I smoke.
............15. No one has the right to say that I shouldn't smoke. The choice should be left up to the individual.

—Lynn Hankins[3]

3. Lynn Hankins, Kent State University, Kent, Ohio. By permission.

SOURCE MATERIALS

Books

AVERY, CURTIS E., and JOHANNIS, THEODORE B., JR. *Love and Marriage.* New York: Harcourt Brace Jovanovich, Inc., 1971.

BAUER, WILLIAM W., et al. *The New Health and Safety.* Glenview, Ill.: Scott, Foresman and Company, 1966.

BURT, JOHN J., and BROWER, LINDA. *Education for Sexuality.* Philadelphia: W. B. Saunders Company, 1970.

CAROLAN, PATRICK J., and FELICE, JOSEPH P. *Tune in to Health.* New York: College Entrance Book Company, 1970.

CORNACCHIA, HAROLD J. *Dimensions in Health: Venereal Diseases.* Chicago: Lyons & Carnahan, 1966.

DIEHL, HAROLD S. *Health and Safety for You.* New York: McGraw-Hill Book Company, 1970.

Dimensions in Health Series: Grades 7-8. Chicago: Lyons & Carnahan.

DOLLOFF, PHYLLIS B., and RESNICK, MIRIAM R. *Patterns of Life: Human Growth and Development.* Columbus, Ohio: Charles E. Merrill Publishing Co., 1972.

GALLAGHER, J. ROSWELL, et al. *Health for Life.* Boston: Ginn and Company, 1964.

GIRDANO, DANIEL A., and GIRDANO, DOROTHY D. *Drug Education: Content and Methods.* Barrington, Illinois: Addison-Wesley Publishing Company, 1972.

JONES, KENNETH L.; SLAINBERG, LOUIS W.; and BYER, CURTIS O. *Consumer Health.* San Francisco: Canfield Press, 1971.

————. *Dimensions.* San Francisco: Canfield Press, 1972.

————. *Drugs and Alcohol.* San Francisco: Canfield Press, 1969.

————. *Sex.* San Francisco: Canfield Press, 1969.

————. *Environmental Health.* San Francisco: Canfield Press, 1971.

KATCHADOURIAN, HERANT, and LUNDE, DONALD T. *Fundamentals of Human Sexuality.* New York: Holt, Rinehart & Winston, 1972.

KIRK, ROBERT H.; MAYSHARK, CYRUS; and HORNSBY, ROBERT PRESTON.
Personal Health in Ecological Perspective. St. Louis: C. V. Mosby,
Co., 1972.

KITZINGER, ANGELA. *Dimensions in Health: Air and Water Pollution.* Chicago: Lyons & Carnahan, 1966.

LAWRENCE, THOMAS G. *Your Health and Safety,* 6th ed. New York: Harcourt, Brace and World, Inc., 1969.

MALFETTI, JAMES L., ed. *Perspectives on Sexuality.* New York: Holt, Rinehart & Winston, Inc., 1972.

MEREDITH, FLORENCE L., et al. *Health and Fitness.* Lexington, Mass.: D.
C. Heath & Company, 1966.

MCCARY, JAMES L. *Human Sexuality.* New York: American Book Company, 1971.

MILLER, BENJAMIN F.; ROSENBERG, EDWARD B.; and STACKOWSKI, BEN-
JAMIN L. *Investigating Your Health.* New York: Houghton Mifflin
Company, 1971.

ODGERS, RUTH F., and WENBERG, BURNESS G., ed. *Introduction to Health
Professions.* St. Louis: C. V. Mosby Co., 1972.

OTTO, JAMES, et al. *Health and Safety for You.* Glenview, Ill.: Scott,
Foresman and Company, 1970.

Ramapo House Health Series: Drugs, Smoking, Alcohol. New York: Ramapo House Educational Publishers, 1970.

RAY, OAKLEY S. *Drugs, Society, Human Behavior.* St. Louis: C. V. Mosby
Co., 1972.

READER'S DIGEST SERVICES, INC., EDUCATIONAL DIVISION. *Life Values
Series.* Pleasantville, N. Y., 1970-72.

RATHBONE, FRANK S., and RATHBONE, ESTELLE. *Health and the Nature of
Man.* New York: McGraw-Hill Book Company, 1971.

SCHNEIDER, ROBERT E. *Health and Growth.* Boston: Allyn & Bacon, Inc.,
1967.

Catalogs

SPENCO MEDICAL CORP., P. O. Box 8113, Waco, Texas 76710. "Education and Gift Catalogue." Smoking, Drugs, V. D.

ELI LILLY AND CO., Audiovisual Film Library, Indianapolis, Ind. 46206.
"Handbook of Audiovisual Services."

AAHPER PUBLICATIONS, American Association for Health, Physical Education and Recreation, 1201 Sixteenth Street, N. W., Washington,
D. C. 20036.

EDUCATIONAL ACTIVITIES, INC., P. O. Box 392, Freeport, N. Y. 11520.
"Classroom Tested Materials."

PHARMACEUTICAL MANUFACTURERS ASSOCIATION, 1155 Fifteenth Street,
N. W., Washington, D. C. 20005.
SEICUS PUBLICATIONS OFFICE, 1855 Broadway, New York, N. Y. 10023.
SCOTT, FORESMAN AND COMPANY, Oakland, N. J. 07436.
CHANNING L. BETE CO., INC., 45 Federal Street, Greenfield, Mass. 01301.

Films

ALFRED HIGGINS PRODUCTIONS, 9100 Sunset Blvd., Los Angeles, Calif.
90069.
AMERICAN CANCER SOCIETY, 219 East 42nd Street, New York, N. Y.
10017.
ASSOCIATION FILMS, INC., 25358 Cypress Avenue, Hayward, Calif. 94544.
C. BAILEY FILM ASSOCIATES, 11559 Santa Monica Boulevard, Los Angeles,
Calif. 90025.
CANADIAN NATIONAL FILM BOARD, 680 5th Avenue, New York, N. Y.
10019.
CATHEDRAL FILMS, INC., 2921 W. Alameda Avenue, Burbank, Calif.
91505.
CHURCHILL FILMS, 6671 Sunset Boulevard, Los Angeles, Calif. 90027.
COLUMBIA UNIVERSITY PRESS (CENTER FOR MASS COMMUNICATION),
562 W. 113 Street, New York, N. Y. 10025.
CORONET INSTRUCTIONAL FILMS, 65 E. South Water Street, Chicago, Ill.
60601.
DENOYER-GEPPERT AUDIO-VISUALS, 5235 Ravenswood Avenue, Chicago,
Ill. 60640.
EALING CORPORATION, 2225 Massachusetts Avenue, Cambridge, Mass.
02140.
ENCYCLOPEDIA BRITANNICA FILMS, INC., 1150 Wilmette Avenue, Wil-
mette, Ill. 60091.
HANK NEWENHOUSE, 1825 Willow Road, Northfield, Ill. 60093.
McGRAW-HILL BOOK COMPANY, INC., 330 W. 42nd Street, New York,
N. Y. 10036.
MODERN TALKING PICTURE SERVICE, INC., 1212 Avenue of the Americas,
New York, N. Y. 10036.
NATIONAL INSTITUTE OF MENTAL HEALTH DRUG COLLECTION, National
Audio-Visual Center, Washington, D. C. 20409.
STERLING EDUCATIONAL FILMS, 241 E. 34th Street, New York, N. Y.
10016.
SOCIETY FOR VISUAL EDUCATION, 1345 Diversey Parkway, Chicago, Ill.
60614.
WALT DISNEY PRODUCTIONS, 800 Senora Avenue, Glendale, Calif. 91201.

Warren Schloat Productions, Inc., 115 Tompkins Avenue, Pleasantville, N. Y. 10570.
Young America Films, 330 W. 42nd Street, New York, N. Y. 10036.

Filmstrips

AAHPER/Publications Sales, NEA Center, Room 627, 1201 16th St.,
N. W., Washington, D. C. 20036.
American Heart Association, 44 East 23rd Street, New York, N. Y.
10010.
Denoyer-Geppert Audio-Visuals, 5235 Ravenswood Avenue, Chicago,
Ill. 60640.
Educational Record Sales, 157 Chambers Street, New York, N. Y.
10007. 1) Human Reproduction, 2) The Dilemma of Drugs.
Encyclopedia Britannica Films, Inc., 1150 Wilmette Avenue, Wil-
mette, Ill. 60091.
Guidance Associates, Subsidiary of Harcourt Brace Jovanovich, Inc.,
Pleasantville, N. Y. 10570.
Hank Newenhouse, 1825 Willow Road, Northfield, Ill. 60093.
Image Publishing Corporation, Dept. KEB, P. O. Box 14, North Sta-
tion, White Plains, N. Y. (Mental Health Series).
Pharmaceutical Manufacturers Assoc., 1155 15th Street, N. W.,
Washington, D. C. 20005.
Popular Science Audio-Visuals, 355 Lexington Avenue, New York,
N. Y. 10017.
Society for Visual Education, Inc., 1345 Diversey Parkway, Chicago,
Ill. 60614.
Time-Life Education, Box 834, Radio City Post Office, New York,
N. Y. 10019.
Westinghouse Learning Press, 100 Park Avenue, New York, N. Y.
10017.
Warren Schloat Productions, Inc., 115 Tomkins Avenue, Pleasant-
ville, N. Y. 10570.
Y.L.P. Materials Corp., Associated Educational Materials Companies,
Inc., Glenwood at Hillsboro Street, Raleigh, N. C. 27600.

Transparencies

Robert J. Brady Company, 130 Q Street, Washington, D. C. 20002.
DCA Educational Products, 4865 Stenton Avenue, Philadelphia, Penn.
19144.
Denoyer-Geppert Audio-Visuals, 5235 Ravenswood Avenue, Chicago,
Ill. 60640.

EDUCATIONAL RECORD SALES, 157 Chambers Street, New York, N. Y. 10007. 1) Special First-aid Problems; 2) Fire Prevention; 3) Common First-Aid Emergencies; 4) Physical Care and Self-Respect; 5) Cell Structure, Function, and Heredity; 6) Growth and the Endocrine Glands; 7) Development Patterns of Pubescent Boys; 8) Development Patterns of Pubescent Girls; 9) The Baby: Its Conception, Growth, and Birth; 10) Development of Concepts and Attitudes; 11) Understanding Venereal Disease.

KNOW: A VISUAL EDUCATIONAL SERVICE, 262 Orinoco Drive, Brightwaters, N. Y. 11718.

RAND MCNALLY AND CO., Box 7600, Chicago, Ill. 60680. (School Department).

3M COMPANY, Visual Products Division, St. Paul, Minn. 55101.

Kits

AMERICAN MEDICAL ASSOCIATION, Department of Health Education, 535 North Dearborn Street, Chicago, Ill. 60610.

THE CREATIVE LEARNING GROUP, A Division of Media Engineering Corporation, 145 Portland Street, Cambridge, Mass. 02139. Drug Educational Package.

CLEVELAND HEALTH MUSEUM, 8911 Euclid Avenue, Cleveland, Ohio 44100. Wonder of Life Birth Models.

FUNCTIONAL RESOURCE UNIT PLAN GUIDESHEET

1. TOPIC: Concept from S.H.E. Study for which the plan is made.
2. GRADE LEVEL: Any specific grade in which the group is interested.
3. TABLE OF CONTENTS (with page numbers).
4. LIST OF GENERAL BEHAVIORAL OBJECTIVES: (Statements involving student behavior that is measurable.) These objectives are to be organized by (1) Cognitive domain; (2) Affective domain; (3) Psychomotor domain.
5. SUGGESTED APPROACHES: These are a series of specific techniques any one of which could be used to pique the interest of the students in the content. They act as an attention getter and are usually used at the beginning of a class. They should take from a few seconds to two or three minutes.
   EXAMPLES:
   1. CONCEPT: Food selection and eating patterns are determined by physical, social, mental, economic, and cultural patterns.
      Have Allen Sherman's record "Why I'm Fat" playing as students come into class. Say, "I'll have to start my diet, tomorrow."
   2. CONCEPT: Use of substances that modify mood and behavior arises from a variety of motivations.
      Take liquor bottle filled with cold tea out of desk drawer and pour into glass. Say, "This class is enough to drive anyone to drink." (Be sure to inform the class before they leave that the contents are tea and not liquor.)
6. CONTENT: Subject matter topics within your concept that are called for by the objectives. Outline form.

7. SUGGESTED LEARNING EXPERIENCES:
    A. Organize according to the type of activity: Values Games, Surveys, Panel Discussions, Small Group Discussions, etc.
    B. Give specific activity listed under the above headings.
    EXAMPLES:
    PANEL DISCUSSIONS:
      1. What do I look for in a date?
      2. What are the problems teenagers face if they marry while still in school?
      3. Whose fault is it if a girl becomes pregnant?
    SKITS:
      1. In a scene with your parents, they have just been told that you had been drinking at last night's party.
      2. You are in the locker room with two friends. One of them offers to supply you with amphetamines.

8. EVALUATION TECHNIQUES:
    A. List different techniques of evaluation to measure the attainment of the General Behavioral Objectives in your plan.
    B. List the techniques under the following categories:
      1. Teacher contrived evaluations
      2. Student self-appraisal
      3. Student evaluation of students
      4. Student evaluation of facilitator
    C. Examples
    Teacher Contrived Evaluations:
      1. Open-ended sentences (Give three or four sentences that fit your concept)
      2. Skits (List some of the criteria that should be included in the completed evaluative tool)

9. TEACHING AIDS AND MATERIALS AVAILABLE:
    A. Films: Rental source, time, color or black and white, cost to rent, brief summary.
    B. Filmstrips: Same information plus number of frames, script or disc, cassette recording.
    C. Pamphlets: Source, address, cost.
    D. Posters: Source, address, cost.
    E. Transparencies: Source, cost, address, titles available.
    F. Models: Source, address, cost.
    G. Kits: Source, address, cost.

    H.   Tapes: Source, address, cost, titles available.

        (Addresses can be listed on one page and coded to save space and typing.)

10. List of agencies, foundations, etc.: Where one can obtain information on topics within your concept.

11. TEACHER REFERENCES: Must be within the last three years for articles; within the last five years for books.

12. STUDENT REFERENCES: Suitable for the grade level to be used as supplementary material for panel discussions, reports, debates, discussions, etc. Same three and five year deadlines apply.

BIBLIOGRAPHY

AMERICAN ASSOCIATION FOR HEALTH, PHYSICAL EDUCATION AND RECREATION, *Health Concepts.* Washington, D. C.: AAHPER Publications, 1967.

BLOOM, BENJAMIN S., ed. *Taxonomy of Educational Objectives: The Classification of Educational Goals,* Handbook I: *Cognitive Domain.* New York: David McKay Co., Inc., 1956.

DALE, EDGAR. *Audiovisual Methods in Teaching,* 3rd ed. New York: Holt, Rinehart & Winston, Inc., 1969.

HARBECK, MARY B. "Instructional Objectives in the Affective Domain." *Educational Technology* 10 (January, 1970): 50.

KRATHWOHL, DAVID R.; BLOOM, BENJAMIN S.; and MASIA, BERTRAM. *Taxonomy of Educational Objectives: The Classification of Educational Goals,* Handbook II: *Affective Domain.* New York: David McKay Co., Inc., 1964.

LESSINGER, LEON M. "Teachers in An Age of Accountability." *Instructor* 80: 10 (June/July, 1971): 19-20.

POSTMAN, NEIL, and WEINGARTNER, CHARLES. *Teaching as a Subversive Activity.* New York: Delacorte Press, 1969.

RATHS, LOUIS; HARMIN, MERRILL; and SIMON, SIDNEY. *Values and Teaching.* Columbus, Ohio: Charles E. Merrill Co., 1966.

ROGERS, CARL R. *On Becoming a Person.* Boston: Houghton Mifflin Co., 1961.

SCHEIN, EDGAR H. *Process Consultation.* Reading, Mass.: Addison-Wesley Co., 1969.

SCHOOL HEALTH EDUCATION STUDY. *Health Education: A Conceptual Approach to Curriculum Design.* St. Paul, Minn.: School Health Education Study, Inc., 1967.

INDEX

Citizen's appeal of, 60
Continuous progress learning, 62-67
Computer assisted instruction, 67-71, 151-156
Computer managed instruction, 71-72
Games as, 54-58
Rank ordering, 56
Table talk, 57
Values continuum, 56-57
Values voting, 54-56
Influences in creating, 75
Instructional materials center, 60-62
Creating one's own, 62
Surveys, original, 72-75
Populations for, 72-73
Utilization of, 73
Lectures, 88-90
Advantages/disadvantages of, 88-89
Modifications of, 90
Lessinger, Leon M., 20
Life styles and:
Attitudes toward patriotic symbols, 10
Behavior, 10-11
Family patterns, 7-8
Language, 9
Male-female family roles, 8
Male-female occupational/recreational roles, 8-9
Personal grooming, 9-10
Religion, 9

M
Male-female occupational/recreational roles, 8
Masia, Bertram, 38-43
Male-female family roles, 8
Media, 104-127
Adhesion boards, 106-108
Dry-mounted materials, 111-112
Films, 122-124
Filmstrips, 121-122
Laminated materials, 112-113
Models, 115-118
Shade charts, 118-119
Slides, 120-121
Suitcase exhibits, 119-120

Tape recordings: reels and cassettes, 115
Tear sheet files, 113-114
Textbooks, 105-106
Transparencies, 109-111
Videotape recorder, 125-128
Models, 115-118
Example of, 116-117

O
Objectives
Behavioral (see also)
Instructional, 37, 38
Learning, 35, 44
Taxonomy of Educational Goals, 38-43
Obsolescence in teaching, 6-7
Open-ended sentences, 3, 132-133

P
Panel discussions, evaluation of, 140-141
Patriotic symbols, attitudes toward, 10
Personal grooming styles, 9-10
Position paper, 133
Postman, Neil, 44-45
Projects, 90-91
Advantages/disadvantages, 90-91
Evaluation of, 142
Modifications, 91
Psychomotor domain, 26, 43-44, 48-49
Behaviors in, 44
Definition of, 43
Development of objectives in, 48-49
Purpose of text, 1, 5

Q
Question and answer, 91-93
Advantages/disadvantages, 92
Modifications, 92-93
Questions
Close-ended, 3
Open-ended, 3, 132-133
Teacher contrived, 83-84, 131-133

R
Rank ordering, 56
Raths, Louis E., 54